THE **MODERN MIDWIFE'S** GUIDE TO

PREGNANCY, BIRTH AND BEYOND

by marie louise

TO MY MUM, DAD, CATHERINE AND JOE. FOR TEACHING ME ALL THAT I COULD LEARN AND BELIEVING IN MY DREAMS.

AND TO MY BETTER HALF, FOR HIS PATIENCE AND UNDERSTANDING OF MY DEDICATION.

THE **MODERN MIDWIFE'S** GUIDE TO

PREGNANCY, BIRTH AND BEYOND

How to have a healthier pregnancy, easier birth and smoother postnatal period

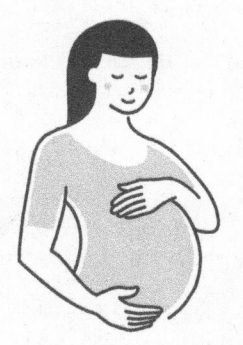

by marie louise

Vermilion
LONDON

3 5 7 9 10 8 6 4 2

Vermilion an imprint of Ebury Publishing,
20 Vauxhall Bridge Road,
London SW1V 2SA

Vermilion is part of the Penguin Random House group of companies
whose addresses can be found at global.penguinrandomhouse.com

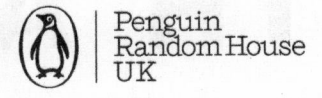

Penguin
Random House
UK

First published by Vermilion in 2020

www.penguin.co.uk

A CIP catalogue record for this book is available from the British Library

ISBN 9781785042966

Typeset in 10/13.5 pt FuturaBT
by Integra Software Services Pvt. Ltd, Pondicherry

Printed and bound in Great Britain by Clays Ltd, Elcograf S.p.A.

MIX
Paper from
responsible sources
FSC® C018179

Penguin Random House is committed to a sustainable future for
our business, our readers and our planet. This book is made from
Forest Stewardship Council® certified paper.

The information in this book has been compiled by way of general guidance in relation
to the specific subjects addressed. It is not a substitute and not to be relied on for medical,
healthcare, pharmaceutical or other professional advice on specific circumstances and
in specific locations. Please consult your GP before changing, stopping or starting any
medical treatment. So far as the author is aware the information given is correct and
up to date as at January 2020. Practice, laws and regulations all change, and the
reader should obtain up-to-date professional advice on any such issues. The author and
publishers disclaim, as far as the law allows, any liability arising directly or indirectly
from the use, or misuse, of the information contained in this book.

CONTENTS

~~~~~

Introduction

AS A MIDWIFE I get asked a lot of questions. Sometimes questions can be answered easily, but often I feel as though we just don't have enough time to really explain everything properly. I hope this book will fill in those gaps, and provide the key information you really need to know about all the common questions that are on most pregnant women's minds. It will also help you go into your midwife appointments feeling like you know what to expect!

My aim is to help you understand and manage each stage of your transition into mumhood so that you can make informed choices every step of the way, understand what is happening in your body, be in control and feel powerful. I want to share with you the most important and amazing things I have learned during my time as a midwife.

Having a baby is hands-down one of the biggest events that will ever happen in your life.

It probably feels as though there is so much you need to know, so many changes going on, and so much to plan for and consider. At times, knowing what's right for you and your baby, planning your birth *and* becoming someone's mum can all be very overwhelming. Know that this is totally normal.

One of the biggest problems for the modern mum is not scarcity of information but actually an information overload. And much of the information we are exposed to, particularly in the media, is not always reliable. The information in this book is based on the latest research and evidence, real mum stories and my years of experience as a midwife working with hundreds of women throughout their pregnancy and birth journeys.

Modern mums are faced with an overwhelming amount of options, opinions and advice, and are asked to make a lot of complex decisions. It can be hard to take it all in and process it. But there's really no rush. Take your time. Read about what you need or want to know in this book when the time feels right for you.

Understanding what really goes on in pregnancy, birth and in those early days as a new mum makes a big difference to how you feel about it. Knowledge is power, after all. How you give birth matters and planning for your time as a postnatal woman will change your entire experience of it. Most people's version of birth is what they see in films and on TV, which generally looks something like this: a woman lying on her back under bright lights screaming, a doctor delivers the baby, she stops screaming and holds the baby wrapped in a towel, everyone smiles.

Birth doesn't usually look like that. We need to create a more realistic – and positive – view of birth.

I hope that *The Modern Midwife's Guide* peels back the layers to help you easily navigate pregnancy, birth and your postnatal period.

MY BACKGROUND

As a child I can remember meeting my siblings for the first time and thinking my mum had this superpower. She could grow people! As I got older and learned that pregnancy is something women have been doing for millennia, I was shocked that this wasn't something I was taught properly about in school. A human can grow another human, inside them? With no instruction? The body does this on its own? I was mind-blown by how the heart, brain and genitals just appear and know what they are meant to do. I once asked my science teacher, 'Isn't that like leaving a load of ingredients in the kitchen and coming home to a baked cake? That can take itself out of the oven?'

My parents and teachers assumed I'd be a teen mum, but I didn't want a baby right then myself; I just had to know more about how humans grow humans. At one point in my teenage years I felt like I was the only person to have all these questions about how we are all here. Until I found midwifery. It was only then that my fascination with pregnancy and birth was satisfied through learning.

But I have to admit I am still disappointed by the serious lack of education surrounding women's health, periods, pregnancy, birth and the postnatal period. This lack of basic yet revolutionary education can lead to women being concerned about things that are normal, and ignoring things that are abnormal. It's vital we all address this with the seriousness it deserves and start talking, educating and sharing information about women's health.

After reading this book I hope you feel how I felt the day I became a midwife. Equipped, still ready to learn, yet also excited about this whole new section in your life.

I want to share with you the most up-to-date evidence and accurate information and hope to give you a few moments of 'oh that makes so much sense ...' and get excited!

You may know me from Instagram or the Modern Midwives and Modern Mums Meet Ups. I wanted to create a community and network for both midwives and mothers on- and offline. I use these platforms for midwives to find like-minded birth experts and for mums to share their stories and talk openly to other mums. As much as I love the digital world and how far you can reach people, nothing really beats communication and face-to-face interaction. So I decided to launch meet up events around the UK.

The Modern Midwives Meet Up launched in February 2019 and has quickly grown into a much bigger national event that I didn't plan for, but I'm grateful to have the opportunity to bring so many birth experts together and talk honestly to improve our practice and therefore the care women receive.

I also thought it was important to bring mums together so they can create their own tribe and build friendships. Loss of identity and loneliness are two common problems new mums face and finding other new mums that share these problems helps to solve them. I often tag mums in my Instagram Sunday

Birth Stories (see page 306) and mums then talk directly to each other and follow each other after seeing that someone had a similar birth or problem to them. We can all learn from, and look after, each other!

HOW TO USE THIS BOOK

To keep it simple I have separated the book into three parts:

- You're Pregnant! Now What?
- Your Positive Birth
- Becoming Mum

At the end of each section I've listed the key points to help summarise the information for you. This will also help you to easily identify what each section is about, so you can dip in and out as you need and go to the sections that are most relevant to you at each stage of your pregnancy – but also feel free to read from page one right through to the end if that is what works best for you!

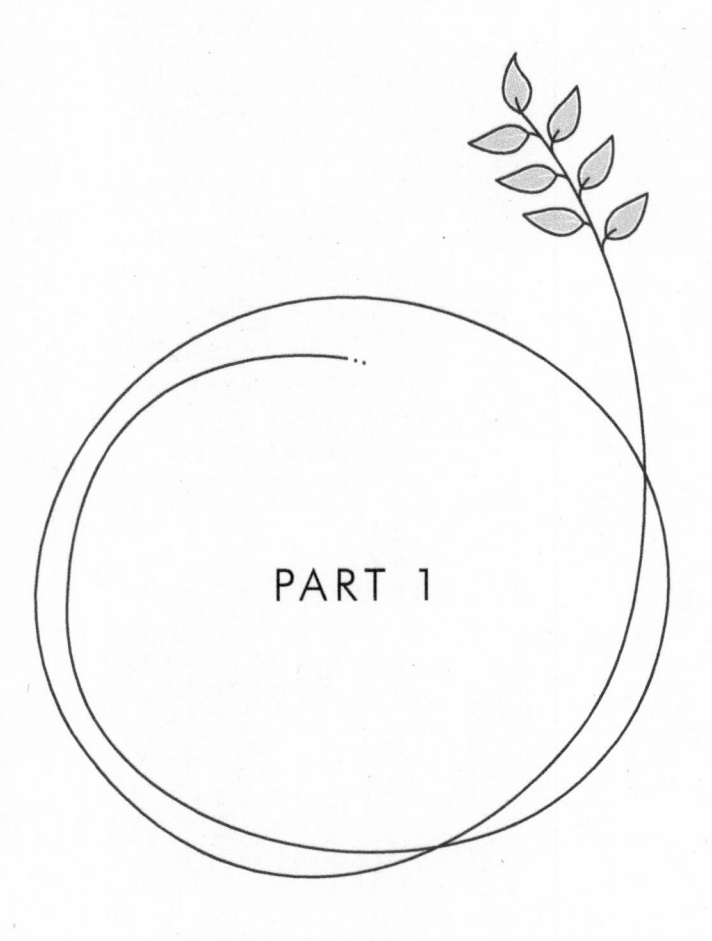

PART 1

You're Pregnant!

Now What?

~~~

Pregnant. That one little word changes your world. Regardless of whether your pregnancy is planned, the unexpected result of one night, or you have had fertility treatment, most women are in shock the moment they find out they are having a baby. 'Oh my god, there's a baby in there!? I'm pregnant ...? Am I really pregnant? Let me just ...'

You may find yourself feeling confused. Maybe you didn't want to be in this position, or maybe you did but now you're not so sure. Maybe you've been trying for such a long time, it seems unreal now that it's actually happened. Or maybe you have started to worry about the fact you got drunk a couple of days ago or that you ate something that isn't recommended in pregnancy.

STOP! Don't beat yourself up, there's nothing you can do about that now, so stop worrying. Millions of healthy babies have been born under exactly these circumstances. Relax and take a breath while you get your head around your news.

No doubt soon though you'll start to wonder 'what do I need to do now?' And if you haven't already, you'll begin wondering if the symptoms you're experiencing are normal. So, we'll start this section by running through the things you need to know in the first instance. Don't worry about the rest for now, there's plenty of time for that. I'll share some handy tips and some fascinating facts about your pregnancy. Then we'll move on to the common concerns most woman have during their pregnancy.

ALWAYS CHECK WITH YOUR MIDWIFE OR GP

The following pages should not be treated as a diagnostic tool. Instead, consider it more of a 'what to expect' guide. Any symptoms or concerns that you have should *always* be checked by your midwife or GP.

THE FIRST THING TO DO

There is something you need to do as soon as you find out you are pregnant; it's not normally spoken about at your first medical appointment, and healthcare professionals sometimes forget to tell you to do this:

Draw an imaginary circle around yourself and promise now to protect, nourish and look after yourself. This is your sacred circle. As hippy dippy as that sounds, it is honestly one of the best things you can do. If you have ever been meaning to start that yoga class (which will now be a yoga for pregnancy class), spend a little more time on self-care, meditate or do more of the things that actually make you happy – now is the time to start. I'm not saying this because I'm a millennial jumping on the self-care band wagon. I'm saying this because, as a midwife, I know just how much of an impact pregnancy has on the mind, body and relationships.

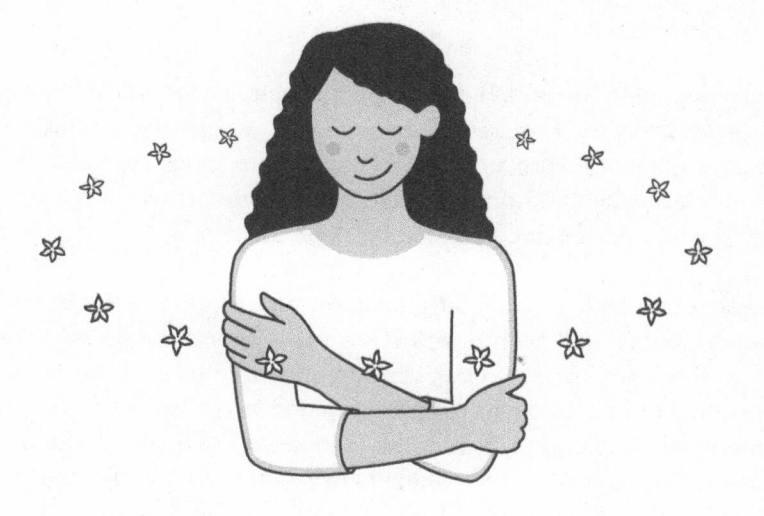

Pregnancy is such unique time in your life, it is important that you give yourself a lot of regard for what your body is doing. Your baby receives cues from you about the outside world and starts to develop their own body and nervous system in response to those cues. We'll go into some more detail about this on page 273 but for now, you, your body and your mind need to come before anything else. It's not easy when you're working, have projects on the go and a social life. But as my nan used to say, 'If you look after the corners, my darling, the middle will look after itself.' Wise old words.

That said, I know how those first few weeks can feel a little stressful and overwhelming at times. Don't worry, these are perfectly normal reactions and you won't be doing your baby any harm; just aim to relax and look after yourself as much as you can.

BOOKING APPOINTMENT

The next thing you need to do is arrange your 'booking appointment'. This is the term we use for the first time you meet your midwife, and it will last for around an hour. You can usually self-refer online these days by using the postcode tool on Find Maternity Services (www.nhs.uk/service-search/other-services/Maternity%20services/LocationSearch/1802).

But traditionally, women booked through their GP and you can still choose this option if you like.

Ideally, you want to be around 8–10 weeks pregnant at your first appointment but it's not a problem if you're further on in your pregnancy. You'll be offered the routine antenatal care and further input from other specialists may be recommended depending on your personal circumstances – we'll cover this fully in 'You're a parent not a patient' on page 32.

Once you're booked, you will be monitored and supported throughout your pregnancy, labour and birth and the postnatal period. While you are in 'a system' you are *not* just a number, you are an individual and you are unique. You are about to embark on the most exciting and incredible journey of your life. As a pregnant woman, you need to be empowered with confidence and self-belief as well as up-to-date knowledge to help you to make informed choices.

MEDICATION

The other important thing to do at this stage is, if you are taking any medication which you think would not be advised in pregnancy, check in with your GP as soon as possible. You can also check BUMPS website (Best Use of Medicines in Pregnancy) as they have a brilliant FAQ section that you may find really useful (www.medicinesinpregnancy.org). Finally, make sure that you are taking 400mcg folic acid supplement or the active form Methylfolate.

For now, those are the only immediate things you need to do.

The normal stuff that happens to your body and how to deal with it

THE HUMAN BODY is one of the most complex organisms on the planet; during pregnancy your entire body is affected! It's amazing to think that there are about seven billion people on the planet and although we are all unique, the way we are grown is the same!

To make room for your growing baby your internal organs need to move and adapt. For example, your stomach, intestines and kidneys will all need to share space with their new neighbours – your baby and placenta.

New hormones quickly appear on the scene, causing changes that can feel a bit chaotic to you. It may not feel like it right now but, I promise, the hormones know what they're doing; they're preparing your body to create the best nest ever. Without any of your conscious control, your hormones have got to work growing your placenta, increasing your flexibility to prepare for birth and stopping your periods – you don't need those right now. You are probably starting to get the picture – and we haven't really scraped the surface yet – that it's totally understandable if you are feeling anything from slightly out-of-sorts to fully derailed.

I have the thickest book ever that runs through each physiological change that occurs during pregnancy, and honestly, it is like reading a science-fiction book. It is *surreal* what your body is doing.

WELCOME TO THE FIRST TRIMESTER

We talk about three trimesters during pregnancy. The first trimester takes you up to 12 weeks, the second trimester is from 13–27 weeks and the third trimester from 28–42 weeks. In this section we will focus on the most common concerns that women have in each trimester.

Finding out you're pregnant can be exciting but you can also have mixed feelings and/or feel worried and nervous; more than 1 in 10 women feel anxious during pregnancy. The cocktail of hormones now pumping through your body may have some effect on your mood. It's easy to blow things out of proportion, especially if you're feeling physically and emotionally tired.

If you feel overwhelmed or feel anxious daily, don't bottle it up – talk to someone you trust, whether it's your partner, midwife or GP. It may also be a good time to start learning and practising yoga breathing techniques to help you to relax. The more you practise these techniques, the easier and more effective they become. This will give you a tool to help you to manage stress or anxiety as well as prepare you for labour and birth. It will be time and effort well invested (see page 115 for yoga in pregnancy).

Morning sickness

Why it's called morning sickness, I don't know. Well I do, as it *is* more common in the morning, but for many of you, it can go on all day. It is often worse first thing in the morning because you've not eaten all night and your blood sugar level has dropped. On a positive note, the hormone hCG (human chorionic gonadotropin) that confirms your pregnancy (in a urine test), is mainly responsible for making you feel sick. Higher levels are actually a sign of a healthy pregnancy. Knowing this may not make you feel better but it may make the sickness feel worth it. That is not to say that if you don't feel sick, something is wrong; generally this means you've just got away with it! Morning sickness is so common that it affects up to 80 per cent of women and can vary in severity from mildly queasy to full-on vomiting.

As morning sickness is so common, the effects of how the nausea and tiredness makes you feel can be dismissed by people around you. It's bloody miserable, I know. Not only that, it's a right nuisance if you've decided not to tell your colleagues you're pregnant but have to swiftly go to the loo or try and pull off the 'peaky look'. If you're really struggling with keeping the secret (and the vomit down) give yourself permission to take a day off and call in sick. Remember your sacred circle.

If you can't keep anything down, you need to see your GP as you might have a condition called hyperemesis gravidarum. Hyperemesis gravidarum can usually be treated with anti-sickness drugs prescribed by your GP, but if it gets out of hand you can become dehydrated and malnourished. For this reason, you will probably need an admission to hospital for a fluid drip and possibly some vitamins. This affects less than 1 per cent of women though.

The good news is if you've got nausea and some vomiting, it usually self-resolves by 16 weeks although some women get it up for up to 20 weeks. That might feel like a lifetime away if you are 10 weeks, so here are some suggestions to help you self-manage until it has subsided:

- Rub fresh lemon peel on your hands as the citrus aroma can really help ward off nausea, especially if other smells set you off.
- Ginger is an age-old natural anti-sickness remedy and is still popular today around the world. Leave a pack of natural ginger biscuits by your bed and nibble on them first thing in the morning to increase your blood sugar levels. Also try fresh ginger tea first thing. If you don't like ginger, try any plain biscuits by the bed and chamomile tea instead.
- Eat little and often – you might not be able to manage full meals, so stock up on snacks like nuts, dried fruit, oat cakes and fresh fruit. Peppermint tea can help to settle your stomach after eating too.
- If you can manage a meal, carbs and starchy foods can help. A plain jacket potato or plain pasta can be easy to eat.
- Fruit and veg smoothies, quickly whizzed up in a blender, can also help you get the nutrition you need if you can't stomach the thought of eating vegetables – this is very common!
- Sip water throughout the day. Some women say even water tastes weird or metallic; a slice of lemon, cucumber or orange in your water bottle can vary the taste.
- Try a wrist acupressure band – many women I have looked after swear by them.

- Fresh air can really help. Simply open the window first thing in the morning and take some slow, nice deep breaths.
- Some women say having someone else prepare their food makes it easier to eat ...
- Try to identify triggers; this is usually a smell or even certain colours can set it off. Then it's easier to avoid them.
- If you have been vomiting, some women like to keep a bag in their handbag so they don't feel stressed about feeling sick in public – dog poo bags work well. Having a sick bag can make you feel less worried about it, and hopefully reduce your stress.

KEEPING YOUR BLOOD
SUGAR LEVELS UP IS ONE
OF THE BEST DEFENCES

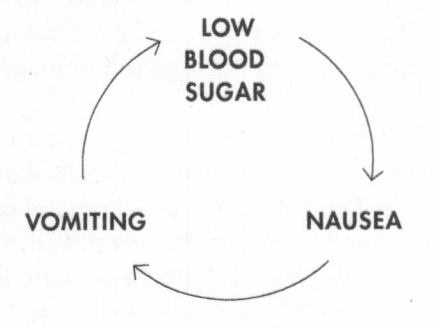

Vomiting and your teeth

I spoke to dentist Jemma Hunter to get some advice about why it is so important to look after your teeth during pregnancy, and we go into this in more detail on page 14.

'If you're frequently being sick it can leave an unpleasant taste in your mouth and can potentially damage your teeth due to the acidity – repeated acid attacks may cause erosion of the surface enamel. Surprisingly, it is not a good idea to brush your teeth straight after vomiting, as the oral environment takes at least 30 minutes to recover to a neutral state; if you brush immediately after vomiting you will be rubbing acid into your teeth. But you can try these options to get rid of that icky taste and help your mouth stabilise after sickness:

- Ideally rinse your mouth with an alcohol-free fluoridated mouthwash.
- If you can't tolerate mouthwash then rinse with plain tap water.
- Use a small dab of toothpaste on your finger and gently smear it over your teeth to get the fresh minty taste without brushing.

Gag reflex

During pregnancy some women develop a heightened gag reflex and you may find yourself retching when trying to brush your teeth, particularly the upper back molars. Of course, you still need to brush your teeth so try:

- Using a toothbrush with a small head – a children's brush will do.
- A 'single tuft' toothbrush can be better for reaching around the back teeth.
- Some people find brushing with warm water helps.
- Take your time – slow down the brushing action and concentrate on your breathing.
- Try other distractions – such as tapping your feet or listening to music.'

Exhaustion

When to comes to coping with exhaustion in the first trimester, remember your sacred circle once again. Try and stay as firmly inside it as possible. Although there will be some things that you *have* to do, anything else can wait or be cancelled – don't feel bad about doing this. If you need to take a nap, order take-out, or eat chips in bed until midday on the weekend, then do it. Lots of women feel the glow in the second trimester – it's coming! – so just take the time out that you need to right now. You'll soon start to feel less exhausted.

It's not surprising that you feel exhausted in your first trimester. Not only is your body growing a baby, you're also growing a whole other organ too: the placenta. By around 12 weeks the placenta has started to function and it takes over the production of the hormones needed for pregnancy. During pregnancy, we focus on growing a baby, but we sometimes forget about one of the most complex and important organs known to the human race. Your placenta acts as your baby's heart, lungs, liver, temperature regulation and so much more. The placenta contains supply lines connecting all of this (technical term is villi) stretching to around 30 miles, and this all has to grow in the first trimester.

Approximately 20 per cent of your blood volume travels to your baby through your placenta. This is also why you are so exhausted – your body is starting to supply a significant amount of blood to a brand-new growing organ.

Once established, your placenta fights off and eliminates pathogens (unwanted intruders) and allows your antibodies to pass through into your baby, building your baby's immune system. The placenta also has the ability to release some of your baby's cells into *your* body in the event that you need repair to any damage to your organs. These cells can stay in your body for decades; this process is called fetal microchimerism. Another sci-fi-like fact that fascinated me was finding out that placental cells can be rather cunning as they disguise themselves as uterine cells in order to trick your uterus so that the placenta can embed itself deep into it and grow your baby. If we knew more about the placenta we would know more about organ transplants, because your placenta is part you and part your baby yet your body doesn't reject it. Such a clever organ! No wonder you feel tired!

Bleeding and spotting

Approximately 20–25 per cent of women experience bleeding or spotting in pregnancy; I have had many tearful phone calls from women thinking the worst. Up to a quarter of women is a lot, so as scary as it can be, try not to panic. Many women also bleed later on in pregnancy; if that does happen it can be for a number of reasons, some more concerning than others. However far along you are you just need to call your midwife or doctor and let them know because you will need to be checked over. If you have a negative blood group and bleed, you may be offered an injection called Anti-D; this neutralises any RhD positive antigens that may have mixed with your blood (so your body won't produce antibodies). If you have a negative blood group you could ask if the non-invasive prenatal testing is available to find out what blood group your baby is.

Constipation

Your digestive system gets sluggish in pregnancy; it goes from a Mercedes on the motorway speed to a coach up a hill. There is a reason for this; the gut slows down so your digestive tract can absorb more nutrients, which is great for growing a baby, but the side effects of this can be constipation and good old heartburn for you – which I will come back to in a moment.

I'm not going to sugar-coat it: constipation is horrible and can go from slightly uncomfortable to quite painful. In order to help your symptoms, you need to work with the new pace of your digestive system. Drink loads of water (two litres per day) and sip little and often throughout the day; this softens things and encourages regular movement. Eat slowly, little and often, and include plenty of wholegrains, veggies, blueberries, beans and add a few dates, figs and chia seeds to your diet.

Listen to your body's cues and try to go as soon as your body is telling you to. I know this is a lot easier said than done sometimes and you can't exactly say to your boss 'sorry, but I need a poo before we start this meeting' (although I wish we were more open in our culture about this). If possible, go as soon as you can when you need to – that email can wait.

Sore and swollen boobs

Sore and swollen boobs can be really uncomfortable in the first trimester. Women often tell me that even the pressure from the water whilst standing in the shower is too much. Your nipples can also get itchy and uncomfortable. This does get a lot better and we will talk about managing your pregnancy boobs further on, but for now wear loose clothing and a comfy bra (see page 18), and swap showers for baths if you can (but don't make them too hot – you'll get hotter quicker in pregnancy and a rise in core body temperature can be dehydrating and make you feel faint.)

Headaches

Headaches are common in early pregnancy and I reckon you can guess why – yup, hormones! Keeping well-hydrated really helps to prevent headaches and paracetamol is thought to be safe to take in pregnancy. Headaches tend to occur less in the second trimester, but you need to let your midwife know if you continue to get them in the second and third trimester because they can be a sign of pre-eclampsia.

THE SECOND AND THIRD TRIMESTER

Here are some of the concerns that women ask me about during their second and third trimester: everyone is different and women get symptoms at different stages, or you may escape them altogether.

Dental dos and don'ts

During pregnancy and after birth it's more important than ever to take care of your teeth, which is why dental care is free under the NHS for pregnant women. While it's not true that a baby steals calcium from your teeth, there are a range of oral conditions, such as inflamed or bleeding gums, that may affect mums-to-be. Book in with your local dentist for a check-up. Although I'm really interested in oral health, I'm not an expert, so I spoke to Jemma Hunter, an NHS family dentist and clinical teacher in paediatric dentistry. She runs an Instagram account @themummydentist and promotes accessible oral health advice for mums and babies. Here's what she told me:

'Maternal oral health is part of overall wellbeing. A baby's milk teeth start to form during the first trimester and their adult teeth begin developing around birth, so taking care of yourself is beneficial to you and your growing baba. It is super-important to visit your dentist during pregnancy, even if you aren't suffering from any of the below symptoms or you haven't been for a while. We can provide routine checks, risk assessment and appropriate advice. There are some aspects of dental care that may alter when you are expecting, such as types of filling material or choosing to delay routine X-rays. We can still safely provide various treatment options, including if you have toothache and require emergency dental work. Your dental maternity exemption then lasts until baby's first birthday, meaning you should also attend appointments after baby arrives so we can assess for any further changes and complete treatment if required. We advise bringing babies along for their first check-up before they turn one too – time for an exciting little family trip to the dentist.

Bleeding gums

This is perhaps one of the most common pregnancy-related dental issues that I get asked about. This is often related to your elevated hormone levels and the slight differences in your immune response whilst pregnant. As bleeding gums can be associated with various conditions like gum disease, infection or inflammation, it's important to see your dentist so they can establish a diagnosis and devise a suitable treatment plan.'

What's that in my knickers?

In traditional Chinese medicine pregnancy is considered a 'damp' condition. This is because increased discharge from your vagina is a common and normal physiological change in pregnancy. The extra discharge is defending your baby and helps prevent any infections travelling from your vagina up to your uterus. However, if you get increased discharge with any itching, pain, a bad smell or stinging/burning on peeing, you need to get it checked out as it could be a yeast infection, bacterial vaginosis or a urinary tract infection – all are common in pregnancy and are easily treated.

Talking of peeing and fluid, you'll need to pee a lot more often during pregnancy. As your baby grows it presses on your bladder. Try not to let this put you off keeping well hydrated; you are more at risk of urine infections in pregnancy and drinking plenty of water to flush out your bladder can really help.

If you feel like you have leaked amniotic fluid, rather than discharge, you need to contact your midwife as soon as possible as there may be a chance that your waters have gone (or 'broken'). Depending on how pregnant you are, your midwife or doctor will make a plan with you about how to manage your waters going.

Skin changes

Some women start to notice skin changes around the second trimester but some don't have any changes at all until the third. Darkening of the skin is very common; this is due to the increase of melanocyte stimulating hormone (MSH) and thought to help darken your nipples so that your baby is able to spot their feeding target better (newborns have poor eyesight at birth). Some women get darker patches on the forehead or cheeks, which can look kind of like a butterfly effect. You may also notice a line down your stomach, called the linea nigra ('black line' in Latin), which is also part of normal skin pigmentation changes.

During pregnancy it is important to make sure you protect your skin from the sun as much as possible. Wear both a hat and a natural sunscreen if you go out in stronger sun, and if you go on a sunny holiday. The darkening of the skin usually subsides and returns to its normal colour about six weeks after birth but in some women the linea nigra is visible up to a year after birth. Whether yours goes or stays it's good to use sunscreen postnatally because darkened skin patches may reappear in the sun.

Hormonal contraceptives, taken after birth, may also create more darkening of the skin. The copper coil (also known as an intrauterine device or IUD) is the only non-hormonal contraceptive available for women at the moment, should you need it.

Stretch marks in pregnancy affect up to 80 per cent of women and can appear in various areas of your body from your tummy to your upper thighs, boobs and even lower back. They usually start to appear or worsen as your pregnancy progresses because of the extra strain on the skin to provide more space. There are a lot of factors involved in why you may or may not get stretch marks, and genetics can really play a part in how your skin adapts and changes in pregnancy. You can't change your genetics but what you can do is work with your body to help prevent them. Here are some top tips:

- Stay hydrated. Water helps skin cells maintain maximum elasticity and suppleness.
- Eat foods rich in vitamin E, zinc and protein that help to repair tissue. For example, almonds, hemp seed, chickpeas and broccoli.
- Dry body brushing increases blood flow to the skin and is a good way to prepare the skin for moisturising. Use a brush designed for the skin and use firm but gentle upward strokes before a shower a few times a week. The brushes with the longer wooden handles are easiest to use. Dry body brushing is more of a preventive measure and you should focus on your legs, upper thighs, bum and arms.
- Moisturise! Body lotions generally have a high water content and lower oil content, whereas oils and balms have the highest oil content. Lotions are probably easier to use daily as they are absorbed quicker and won't leave marks on your clothes. Oils and balms are best in the evening as they can soak into the skin overnight and it won't matter too much if they get on your PJs. Rosehip oil is expensive but it's good for scars and stretchmark prevention. If it is hard to reach some areas later on in pregnancy try spraying on oil – you can put the oil of your choice in a refill spray bottles. Or if you have a partner, ask them massage it in for you.

Even after doing all of these you may still get stretch marks and some women get quite upset about them. Please remember how normal and common it is. For years women have felt the need to hide their very normal and beautiful postpartum bodies, but now there is a huge positive movement online, and it's about time, to help normalise the reality of women's bodies. Stretch marks are nothing to be ashamed of and are very normal for most women that have had babies. The problem is that we have all been sold the wrong idea of what is normal.

Haemorrhoids (piles)

These irritating little things can be brought on due to increased blood flow and the gradually increasing weight of your baby putting pressure on your pelvic floor and back passage. You can help to prevent haemorrhoids by eating a diet high in fibre – going easily prevents you straining on the loo, which can make things worse.

My friend cycles a lot and she told me about a pre-cycle trick she uses so she doesn't have to worry about finding a loo out on a long bike ride. She drinks a pint of water and an hour later she sits on the loo and gently rocks backwards and forwards (no straining), just rocking, and it makes her go. I haven't found any reliable medical research to support this but there is no harm in water and gentle rocking; why not try it?

You can also buy haemorrhoid creams but speak to a pharmacist first about what they recommend for pregnant women.

Heartburn

As your baby grows there is less room in your body for daily digestion. As previously mentioned, your gut has also slowed. You also have a ring of muscle (oesophageal sphincter) that relaxes during pregnancy, which can allow acid to leak back up. This can all cause heartburn, which can be rather unpleasant! You can help reduce the acidity naturally with diet – as mentioned before, try to eat little and often rather than bigger meals. Food containing high amounts of saturated fat are the most commonly reported triggers for heartburn, alongside spicy food and acidic drinks like orange juice.

Be conscious of your position while eating too; try to sit upright to take pressure off your stomach and avoid eating a meal less than two hours before bed. Some herbal teas may help, such a ginger or chamomile. Gaviscon Original is safe to take in pregnancy, so if it's bothering you most around bedtime, have a bottle at arm's reach so you can grab it without having to getting up in the night. You can also request medication from your GP if it is severe and none of the above helps.

Pregnancy boob job

Pregnancy gives most women a free boob enhancement. If you are already naturally well enhanced, you may find your boobs have become rather heavy. By late pregnancy your bra size can go up by a whopping three sizes. Some women love it and it makes them feel sexier than ever and other women don't welcome the changes or find it uncomfortable. Either way, you do need to pay a little bit of attention to your new boobs.

It's best to avoid underwired bras because they can dig into your boobs, pressing on tissue that needs to be freely able to adapt, and can potentially block milk ducts. There are loads of maternity bras on the market and some are rather expensive (you don't necessarily need the most expensive one); bear in mind that boob changes will continue throughout your pregnancy so you might need to buy a couple. Sometimes just a 'giving' yet supportive sports bra can work well for the first few months. Depending on whether or not you breastfeed, changes to your boobs will continue on into breastfeeding and beyond. If you plan to breastfeed, consider getting a breastfeeding bra in late pregnancy; it is a good idea to get some practice using it because it can be really frustrating when your baby is crying and you need to feed but you are fiddling around with the little clips trying to get it undone.

Breastfeeding bras need to be non-wired, non-padded, adjustable and with the drop-down cup. Quite a few shops do free bra fittings so take advantage of this and make sure you get the best fitting bra for you.

Dizziness

A lot of women feel slightly dizzy or faint during pregnancy and there are a few different reasons why, such as a drop in blood pressure, hormones, being overheated or anaemia (low iron levels). If you are feeling dizzy it is always worth mentioning to your midwife as you can get a blood test to check what is going on. To help dizziness:

- Get up slowly after sitting or lying down.
- As soon as you feel faint sit down quickly.

- Avoid lying on your back. This can be tricky at night, but for tips on this see page 20.
- Stay hydrated and make sure you are drinking plenty of water.

Feeling sweaty

Your body pumps more blood during pregnancy (up to 50 per cent more) and the combination of that along with hormonal fluctuations can make you feel unbearably hot and sweaty. You might want to get a desk fan for work and for your bedroom. Try wearing layers of natural fibres such as cotton so you can easily take them on and off as the sweats come and go. If you can afford to, invest in some maternity clothes for maximum comfort throughout the second and third trimesters – the extra elastic and comfort does make a difference. There are some amazing second-hand clothes out there, too, which is also an eco-choice.

Sleep struggles

Usually the struggle to get to sleep starts towards the end of the second, and beginning of the third, trimester. You need to do all you can to help your body switch off, relax and sleep. The first thing is to try to avoid using your phone, iPad, laptop etc. at least an hour before bed. The blue light coming from electrical devices can stimulate us and mess with our sleep rhythms, keeping us awake.

Make sure your bedroom is designed for sleep. Make it as dark as possible, and use blackout blinds or an eye mask if you are being woken by light coming in. Feeling hot during the night sometimes wakes women up too. Try making your room slightly cooler than usual (open a window if you can) as this may help you sleep through the night, which is a major achievement in mid- to late-pregnancy.

Try a simple bedtime routine to help your body and mind wind down, helping you get off to sleep. Try a bath with lavender oil in it, a simple breathing exercise, and listening to a hypnobirthing CD (if this is something you decide to do see page 182 for more on hypnobirthing). Whatever you decide to include in your routine be consistent with it; eventually your mind should get used to it, making sleep easier.

Needing to wee is one of the most common reasons women either struggle to get off to sleep or wake up in the night. Keep well hydrated throughout the day but try not to drink two hours before bedtime – especially diuretics (wee enhancers) like tea and coffee, even if they are decaf. More liquid in, the more liquid out. On that note, avoid caffeine in the afternoon because it can stay in your system for 6–10 hours (depending on genetics and metabolism), so check the time before you opt for a coffee.

Pregnancy pillows can help you feel comfortable and are worth investing in. There are plenty on the market and if you chose a versatile one it can come in handy for breastfeeding too.

The press put out some lovely 'clickbait' for pregnant women a little while ago about how the risk of stillbirth increases if you don't sleep on your left. I had women setting alarms throughout the night to make sure they were sleeping on their left ... Although it is true that it is best to sleep on your left side because the blood flows easier that way, your right is fine if it's more comfortable. Avoid sleeping on your back as this can restrict blood flow to you and your baby. If you wake up on your back, don't panic, just roll over onto your side again.

Some pregnant women have weird or vivid dreams. This is due to hormonal changes and your emotional processing: you and your body are going through a lot of changes and sometimes it's reflected in your dreams. No matter how weird and wonderful they are, don't worry – it's your mind's way of coping with your thoughts throughout the day and dreaming about an ex doesn't mean you still have feelings for them!

Insomnia

We'll go on to talk more about brain changes in a minute, but towards the end of pregnancy you are in a heightened state of awareness and this can also affect your sleep patterns. In late pregnancy, you may well find yourself feeling fidgety with expectation, impatience and frustration at feeling uncomfortable, and general restlessness.

Nap during the day if you can, and don't you go feeling bad about this. I am a big fan of naps and I encourage mums to work them into their day, especially later on in pregnancy. The Healthy Baby Cohort Study in China (2012–2014) found that: 'Afternoon napping and frequency of afternoon napping during late pregnancy were associated with a reduced risk of low birth weight babies.'

So, what I'd take from this study is that napping is probably very good for your baby too.

Napping has a range of health benefits for you, even if you don't have insomnia; they can help to improve mood, alertness and overall performance. If you get napping, you're in good company; Albert Einstein, Winston Churchill and his wife, and John F. Kennedy are all known to have taken regular afternoon naps. Plus, if you aren't good at napping it's an opportunity to master the skill, one that will come in handy in those early newborn days when most parents survive on naps after many broken nights of sleep.

There are a few types of naps:

- Planned nap – for example, preparation for if you want to stay up later in the evening.
- Emergency nap – you're exhausted and have to stop for a nap.
- Habitual nap – which you take around the same time each day.

Your nap will reflect your lifestyle and whether or not you've started maternity leave, for example, as you can be more flexible at this time.

For most people, the best time for a day time nap is around 2pm after lunch when your blood sugar is stable; if you nap too late in the afternoon it may interfere with your night-time sleep. Napping is also an individual thing, so a bit of trial and error might be needed.

To help with relaxation and getting off to sleep, and if you have the budget for it, you could try reflexology; so many women say that it's a game-changer. Opt for someone that specialises in pregnancy; The Association of Reflexologists website can point you in the right direction for your local reflexologist specialising in pregnancy, who will be qualified and insured.

Brain changes

As with every part of your body, your brain also goes through changes during pregnancy. Your brain is changing and new circuits are forming, so don't be surprised if you're a bit forgetful or struggling with stuff that you normally 'get on with'. Science is only just uncovering the huge changes your brain goes through. Researchers in Barcelona and Leiden Universities scanned pre-

pregnant and postnatal women's brains. They found that pregnancy alters and fine-tunes the outer layer of grey matter in the brain. From the brain scans *alone* it was possible for the researchers to pick out women who had had babies. Women who experienced the most brain changes reported strong bonds with their babies; researchers and neuroscientists believe this is because they are more sensitive to their baby's facial expressions, hands and smell. More research into the effects of these changes is needed to be clear on this though.

It's worth knowing that research about the pregnancy brain shows that the changes have no overall effect on work performance and can even help you with decision-making as your brain is becoming fine-tuned to better read the facial expressions and body language of your colleagues or clients. It is thought that you become more in tune in order to be more attentive. If you're a first-time mum these changes are more significant as the circuitry is being set up – you are evolving into a mum.

In the third trimester, the part of the brain that is responsible for recognising and responding to fear (the amygdala) is sensitised to help us have a heightened awareness and our threat response is activated. This is so that you can look after yourself and your baby – it's an evolutionary defence mechanism. If you have a family pet and she becomes a mum, you may find that she changes and responds differently or becomes stressed if you go near her newborn babies – this is the amygdala at work. And humans are similar!

Braxton Hicks

Named after a British gynaecologist, John Braxton Hicks, these irregular tightenings can be felt from as early as 24 weeks, especially if you have been pregnant before. You probably won't be aware of them so early in your first pregnancy though. They are just practice runs for labour and are thought to also help with toning the walls of your uterus. They tend to start during physical activity, at end of the day, after sex or when you're dehydrated.

Lasting about 30 to 60 seconds, the tightening begins at the top of your uterus and gradually spreads down. They're not painful and are perfectly normal. Don't worry if you don't feel any Braxton Hicks as not all women do. If they are painful and regular then they are possibly not Braxton Hicks and are more like real labour – time to call your midwife.

Diastasis recti

It's common for the two muscles that run down the middle of your stomach to separate during pregnancy; this is called 'diastasis recti' (a lot of medical words are Latin-derived). The amount of separation varies and can increase if you are having twins and usually with the more babies you have. It happens because your uterus pushes the muscles apart, making them a bit longer and weaker. There is a lot that you can do postnatally to help bring them back together, but during pregnancy is it important to prevent the separation from getting worse, so avoid doing crunches or sudden sitting-up movements during the second and third trimesters. Getting out of bed by rolling onto your side rather than sitting upright also helps to protect your muscles. You do not want to do any sudden movements that require you to isolate the abdominal muscles anyway.

Pelvic girdle pain (PGP)

Pelvic girdle pain affects about one in five women and it is an umbrella term for pain surrounding the entire pelvic region. The pain tends to increase towards the end of the second trimester and into the third due to the increasing weight of your baby.

Unfortunately, because PGP is caused by pregnancy hormonal changes, ligament and skeletal changes and the weight of your baby, the main cure for PGP is having the baby. The good news is that pain resolves after birth for most women and there are ways you can prevent and manage it.

Some women start to experience symptoms as early as 24 weeks and if that is you, then it is important to see a specialist women's health physiotherapist as soon as possible. They can provide you with tailored exercises and manual therapy techniques to help relieve symptoms. They can also advise on other management strategies such as a maternity belt or taping for support. It's not a one-rule-fits-all with PGP so you need to get specialised advice if it's come on early and is worsening quickly. Your GP or midwife can refer you to a specialist on the NHS; do try to get in early as there is often a waiting list.

Lastly, doctors can prescribe pain relief but bear in mind that these are often opioid-based and will cross the placenta, so your baby will get a bit of the drug. If you are taking opioid-based painkillers for an extended period of time your baby may need to be monitored after birth as they can be affected by this. The Royal College of Obstetricians and Gynaecologists (RCOG) recommend that the lowest doses of opioids should be taken for the shortest time possible.

To help prevent you manage any PGP and reduce the need for painkillers, there are some really simple things you can do listed below – the difficult part is remembering to do them as most of us are creatures of habit:

- Avoid standing on one leg e.g., sit down to put on trousers.
- Avoid heavy lifting or twisting.
- Try to keep knees together when rolling in bed.
- Keep weight even on both legs when standing and when getting up from a chair.
- Sleep with a pillow between the knees (if you're lying on your side) to keep hip and knee in line.

If you have a job where you are sitting down most of the day, it is important to get up every hour and walk around to help release any tension and keep your joints lubricated. If you work for a company, it's worth asking if they will get you a chair or coccyx wedge to support your lower back. If you work from home have a look at your options online; they aren't too pricey but can make a big difference to your posture and therefore your pain.

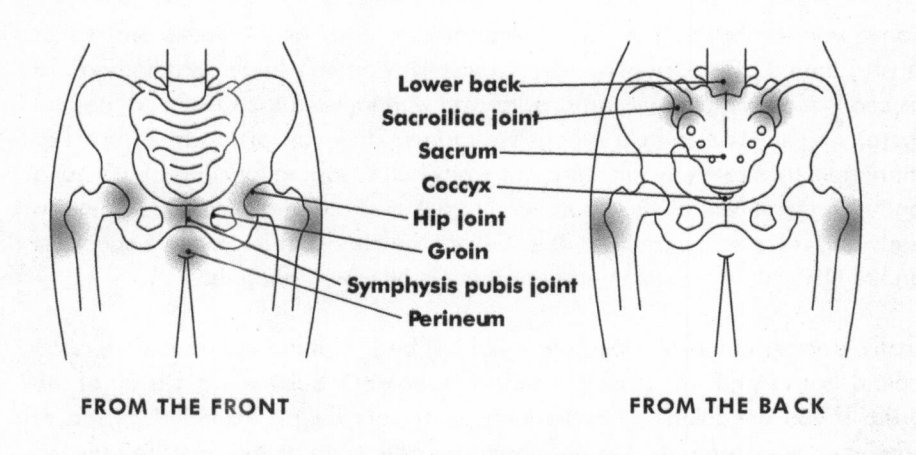

Lower back
Sacroiliac joint
Sacrum
Coccyx
Hip joint
Groin
Symphysis pubis joint
Perineum

FROM THE FRONT   **FROM THE BACK**

Another thing that I find helps women who drive or who have a long commute is the bin-bag trick – glamorous I know. Pop a plastic bin bag on your seat so you can keep your legs together as you get into the car, and then swing around smoothly, rather than have to keep opening your pelvis and unevenly distributing weight. Making little things easier each day and being gentle with your body can help you avoid a future build-up of pain.

POSTURE DURING PREGNANCY

Your centre of gravity and posture change during pregnancy due to your increasing bump. Posture matters in pregnancy as your changing body will impact on your centre of gravity; some women say that they become clumsy and slightly off balance, so it's a good idea to think about your footwear (wearing supportive shoes etc.) and to be aware of your posture. Poor posture may lead to back pain too, so here are a few things to think about:

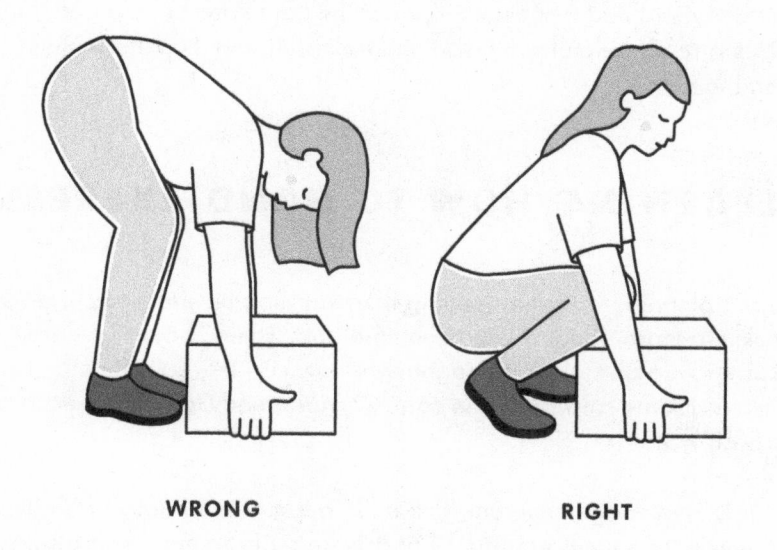

WRONG   RIGHT

- Stand tall is the general rule. If you stand and walk tall, you'll feel more stable and less tired.
- Avoid hollowing or arching the small of your back as you stand or sit. Instead, lengthen your lower back downwards and feel how your

tailbone is slightly tucked under. Get into the habit of keeping your pelvis tilted like this and this will encourage your baby to move into the optimal fetal position (OFP).

- When lifting or bending, imagine you have a hinge at your hips and let your knees bend. Let your legs do the work rather than your back.
- Avoid slouching. Use an upright chair that supports your spine and make it comfortable with cushions to support you. Slumping into the sofa may be comfortable to start with but as your bump grows, you will need to think about keeping your hips higher than your knees, to encourage baby into the OFP for birth (see above).
- When sitting, keep your feet flat on the ground. Switch chairs if you need to, or put your feet on a book.
- Sit upright when driving and use a wedge or cushions to keep your hips higher than your knees.
- Don't cross your legs when seated.
- Later in pregnancy, lie on your side (preferably left) with a pillow under your head and another under the bent knee of your upper leg. This is really helpful when you find it difficult to get comfortable in bed too.

LEARNING HOW TO HAND-EXPRESS

If you are planning on breastfeeding then learning how to hand-express is a great skill to learn about if you have time now. There is a lot going on when baby arrives, so giving this some thought now can be really helpful. You can even harvest some colostrum (see page 27) now, ready to have an extra supply if you baby needs it.

Your body is making colostrum (first milk, a.k.a. 'liquid gold') from as early as 16 weeks in your pregnancy, but it is not safe to start hand-expressing until you are 36 weeks because it is thought that breast stimulation may help to bring labour on. Colostrum is packed with infection-fighting properties (see page 288). Having your own mini milk supply at the ready before baby arrives is great if your baby doesn't breastfeed well in the first few days, is a little sleepy, or if you are taking beta blockers to control high blood pressure.

You can also give your baby your own milk to help prevent or treat things like low blood sugar or jaundice. Women with diabetes are often advised to 'harvest colostrum' because their babies are more at risk of having low blood sugar, but the benefits of just knowing how to do this ahead of time will help most women as you will have enough to learn and do when your newborn arrives.

A note for diabetic mums: controlling and stabilising your blood sugars in pregnancy is vital for optimum health for both you and your baby. It will reduce the risk of you becoming unwell and reduce the risk of your baby having low BMs after birth and needing further input.

Some hospitals have a policy especially for antenatal expression; your midwife should be able to give you small sterile bottles, syringes or other containers with ID labels to save your colostrum if you want to give it a go. You can then freeze and store it at home, and your midwife will advise you on this.

When I say mini milk supply, I really mean mini. Getting 1ml of colostrum is a massive achievement. A newborn baby will usually only need a few millilitres of colostrum for a satisfying first feed. If you hand-express regularly, about three times a day, you will start to build more of a milk supply. You only need to do this for five minutes; go easy and be gentle on yourself.

If you are at risk of pre-term labour or have other complications (like a cervical suture in place) it may not be safe to do this so talk to your midwife first.

How to express colostrum
It is worth getting the hang of expressing colostrum even before baby arrives (see page 26). If you try expressing and nothing comes out, please don't worry. This can happen and not everyone is able to get milk out during pregnancy, on the other hand, some women leak milk in pregnancy; both are normal.

Simply having read this and knowing how to hand-express may help once your baby has arrived.

1. Make sure you've got clean hands. You will need to have a sterile syringe ready (as mentioned, your midwife should be able to give this to you).

2. Get warm, comfy and relaxed; maybe have a bath or pop a warm flannel on your breasts.
3. Give yourself a gentle massage to help milk flow.
4. Create a 'C' shape around the nipple with four fingers under the breast and the thumb towards the top. Your thumb and fingers should be about 2–3cm away from the base area around the nipple (don't squeeze your nipple)
5. Use your thumb and index finger to gently squeeze. Release the pressure and then repeat, creating a rhythm. This should *not* hurt. Try not to slide your fingers over your skin as this can cause bruising and pain. If the colostrum doesn't come out, try moving your fingers slightly closer to your nipple or further away; it may take a little bit of experimenting to find where's best for you, we all have different sized nipples and areola, get to know your own anatomy.
6. Collect your colostrum with the sterile syringe. Colostrum is really concentrated and will usually come out of drop by drop. At first, you may only get a few drops, but with practice and time, you should get more.
7. When the drops start to slow down, move your fingers around to try a different section of your breast but make sure you are still a little way from your nipple.
8. When the flow from one breast has slowed, swap to the other breast.

REMEMBER, YOU ARE NOT ALONE

Although at times the symptoms of pregnancy can may make you feel like you are alone in what you are going through, remember, you are never really alone. Millions of women have felt how you do right now. Midwives, doctors, yoga teachers, physiotherapists, friends and family are all there for you. Also, your baby is with you all the time. You are never really alone.

As difficult as some of these symptoms can be to deal with, also remember that by the end of your pregnancy your body has achieved incredible things to grow your baby. Your bladder has become a trampoline (as your baby's head is bouncing around on it), your lungs have changed shape, your boobs have started making milk, your blood volumes has increased by up to 50 per cent and that's just the tip of the iceberg. Scientists have been able to create machines and replicate just about anything, but no one has ever been able to invent a fully functioning womb because it's so sophisticated and complicated. Incubators are the closest thing we have but they aren't a patch on you.

KEY POINTS

- Remember, you're not just growing a baby, you're also growing an incredibly complex and unique organ, the placenta, too!
- Remember your sacred circle and do what you need to get by.
- You may experience various symptoms in pregnancy but your body is growing another human and needs to make a lot of changes – it knows what it is doing.
- Your brain changes significantly so you can respond better to your baby's cues.
- You're not alone – there are a range of experts, midwives and doctors to help advise you.

YOGA BREATHING IN PREGNANCY

Yoga breathing can be done anywhere and any time you need or want to relax. If you can find a quiet place, this is ideal but don't worry if you can't, just do the best you can. The practice can be done lying down in early pregnancy but when you get to around 20 weeks, make it a sitting practice as the weight of the baby can interfere with your circulation when in a lying position. You can do this during a break at work, while waiting at an appointment, or at home before sleeping. Using yoga breathing can help with insomnia, nervousness and encourages the body to calm down, leading to a calmer and clearer mindset. The entire body is affected by simply breathing mindfully.

My mum Julie is a yoga for pregnancy teacher, and has been practising yoga for over 30 years; she has taught me a lot about using yoga to relax and manage times of personal difficulty, change or self-doubt, and she helped me write this section. You can use these breathing techniques anytime during pregnancy or add them to your bedtime routine – whatever works for you.

Yogic breathing simply involves deep, comfortable breaths:

• The in-breath is slow, smooth and deep. Begin with the breath in the abdomen then feel the chest starting to expand outwards and upwards; keep feeling it right up to the top of the lungs.

- Allow the out-breath to be equally smooth and slow.
- Continue with a few more in and out breaths (or 'rounds' or 'cycles') until you feel the pattern of your breath has become like the swell of the sea. Do not strain or try too hard; stay relaxed throughout.

LENGTHENING THE OUT-BREATH

This very simple technique is great for relaxation. All you are aiming to do is to make your out-breath longer than your in-breath. Lying or sitting, take your awareness to your breathing without trying to change it or make any judgement. Keep the awareness for a couple of minutes then begin to make your out-breath slightly longer. Continue to lengthen the out-breath and before you know it, the in-breath has also become longer. Your breathing will have become slower, smoother and more relaxed. Keep your awareness on your breathing and if your mind wanders, try saying mentally:

'I am breathing in ... I am breathing out ... I am breathing in ... I am breathing out'. Start by practising this for about 10 minutes each day, preferably in the morning before you start your day. If you can't practise in the morning, set aside some time somewhere in your day or evening to do this. If you are able to extend your practice to 15–20 minutes, it will become a useful part of your routine and your baby will also really enjoy the benefits of your relaxation time.

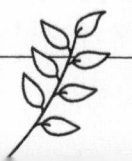

You're a parent not a patient

AS YOU NOW know about some of the expected changes pregnancy can bring about, it is the perfect time to tell you a bit more about what to expect from healthcare professionals, the different types of care you may be offered, and how to make informed choices. We will also touch on making the most out of your appointments so you can really get what you need out of the care you receive.

At a time when you're feeling a bit vulnerable or nervous about what is to come, you might not feel like you have the power, strength or knowledge to call the shots. But one of the most important things you need to know is that you *always* have a choice. No one can tell you what to do. This is about your body, your health, your wellbeing, your baby and your circumstances. All of these are unique to you. Others may offer advice, some of which is priceless (and some of which is useless), but no one can tell you what to do. There will be lots of decisions to make along the way, so this section focuses on what to expect and how to navigate your decision-making in the care of maternity experts.

You are the boss and you call the shots. Every. Single. Time.

APPOINTMENTS AND ROUTINE TESTS

Every pregnant woman at every appointment will have a decision to make about something. For example, tests, antenatal checks and screenings are all part of the UK's routine maternity care pathway. You'll be offered things like blood tests, BMI measurement, two scans (usually a combined or dating scan around 12 weeks, which estimates your due date and screens for Down's syndrome and another one around 18–20 weeks to check for abnormalities, you'll also be able to find out the sex of your baby at this scan if you want to), carbon monoxide testing – even if you don't smoke – testing your wee, measuring your bump and listening to your baby's heartbeat. A quick aside: many women ask what does 'FHHR' on their notes mean? It stands for 'fetal heart heard and regular' and it's normal.

Most women are happy to have all the routine tests on offer but each test is still a choice and you don't have to have anything you don't want. You can ask for more information before making any decision. The NHS offers these routine tests and screening to all women because they help to keep an eye on your baby's development, and to see how your body is coping with the vast changes and new demands pregnancy asks of it. You are perfectly capable of adapting to the physical changes but for some women these increased demands can cause other conditions, and that's when we recommend further testing, referral to an obstetric doctor or another specialist.

Many women don't need further tests beyond the routine tests; we consider you to be 'low risk' and midwives can provide all the care you need. We call this 'midwifery-led care'. Even if you have more tests, if they come back as normal (this happens all the time) you're still considered to be 'low risk'.

MEASURING YOUR BABY'S WEIGHT

A lot of women I meet become concerned about their baby's weight because (if you consent to it) we now measure all baby's growth more closely. We use a customised growth chart going by your ethnic origin, height, weight and information about any previous babies. The chart has a few lines predicting how your baby will grow. At about 25 weeks, and at each appointment after that, we measure your tummy and plot it on your graph. Sometimes the measurement is slightly outside, either above or below, the predicted inclining line of growth. This can be worrying to mums as it can sometimes look like your baby has lost weight or has suddenly had a huge growth spurt. As hard as it is, please try not to worry too much about the plots outside the graph. I speak to many women that are so worried about these 'off' readings. Because this one reading alone isn't always accurate, if we think your baby needs extra scans to check their growth, we will arrange these with you. Also (more often than not) the scans come back as being normal anyway.

Some women may be offered closer monitoring or perhaps medication for different conditions. This is when the routine care pathway changes from 'low risk' and moves into 'high risk' so a doctor will need to take over your care plan. You'll still see a midwife, but the lead professional will become a doctor and this is known as 'obstetrics-led care'.

Please don't worry if that's you. Obstetrics-led care or 'high risk' is a fairly broad-spectrum term that is used for a wide variety of conditions. It's more of a heads-up to doctors and midwives than it is a label for you to carry around.

Making the most of your antenatal appointments

Whatever care pathway you're on (midwife-led or doctor-led), at some point most women will be seen by a midwife for some of the routine and other antenatal appointments. You should be given an outline of your routine appointments so you know when you need to be seen and what to expect at that appointment.

Most first-time mums have about ten routine appointments plus two scans. If you have had a baby before, you'll usually be offered slightly fewer appointments, usually seven plus two scans. We always want to test your wee at these appointments. You'll be surprised at the amount of information we get from your wee. From possibly needing a diabetes check to infection and even organ dysfunction – we can identify a lot. So, unless you are doing your pee sample at home and bringing it in, come to your appointment needing to pee (not hard when you're pregnant, I know, but I have had to wait for women to go to the loo so I can complete their antenatal check). By knowing what to expect at each appointment you can prepare yourself better. If you have any non-urgent questions that pop up, start a little log on your phone now so that you don't forget.

As you now know you'll be offered tests in each antenatal appointment. If you have chosen to take them, midwives need to make sure we complete all of the tests properly and document them, and this takes up the majority of the time. If you have questions or anything you'd like to run through, it is really helpful to let us know at the beginning of the appointment. This allows us to plan for your needs properly and we can sometimes ask a maternity support worker or student to do some of those tests while we address your other questions or needs.

Sometimes you can tell us of any queries before, at an earlier appointment, or call ahead and let us know. For example, I didn't have a particularly busy clinic one day but I knew I had three women who would need some extra time, so that morning I asked if a third-year (almost qualified) student midwife could work with me. That way she was able to learn and help by doing the majority of the tests while I could really address the concerns of those women who needed me. It worked out perfectly. The student learnt a lot, the women left feeling confident and cared for, and I left knowing I'd done my job well. Winning! Had I not known that in advance I would have offered for the student midwife to work with someone else – as I had a quieter clinic – and had less time for those women that needed more advice.

Information overload

There's usually a wide range of answers to questions you have throughout pregnancy and new information, policies and research is ever evolving and emerging. Some women have told me that they find this confusing, intimidating or overwhelming. Knowing how to think critically about the answers you get and accept early on that there probably isn't one solution to your circumstance can be helpful.

There will be a range of answers to your questions and you can find what works for you somewhere in that range. There's no blueprint to get from pregnancy to motherhood and there's no one way to become a mother: everyone is different.

If you're diagnosed with anything during or after your pregnancy you will need to ask questions so you can think critically about your choices.

For example, try these questions:

- 'What is ...?'
- 'How can this affect me and my baby ...?'
- 'What does this diagnosis mean for me personally moving forward ...?'

These simple questions can help you connect the information based on your personal circumstance and process it properly. Never be afraid to ask all the questions you need to, because your confidence and understanding are key to reducing anxiety and fear.

KNOWING YOUR RIGHTS

~~~~

Whether you are low or high risk, you'll need to make many choices throughout your pregnancy, birth and beyond. All healthcare professionals know that you make the final call, but sometimes women feel as though they are in a 'system' of care rather than at the centre of their own individual care.

Catharina Schram is a Consultant Obstetrician and trustee of the Birth Rights Organisation. She does a lot of work around informed consent and protection of women's birth rights, and is a true advocate for women when it comes to promoting informed choice and informed consent. I asked if she could give one message to all women about their choices and consent, what would it be? She said:

'When it comes to a decision about any medical treatment, investigation, procedures, intervention or non-intervention in childbirth, the decision lies with the woman. The role of the healthcare practitioner is to maintain a dialogue with the woman (and her family as appropriate), that helps determine what information the woman wants and needs, and providing that information in an unbiased way. Ultimately that dialogue will help her achieve an informed choice. Critically, the woman is the decision-maker.'

Healthcare professionals want to advocate choice, but I can't turn a blind eye to the times women have told me that they feel they don't have choices, and are in a system. If at any point you feel like the decision-making isn't being explained, then it's really important to speak up and say how you feel. You could even use these words: 'I don't feel like I'm making an informed decision. Using the latest evidence please can you explain ...' which may help you get the information you need to move forward with *your* decision.

'Policies, guidelines and standard operating procedures have been introduced in their hundreds. The goal? To create a practice that was standardised and evidence-based, to reduce risk and improve safety. The difficulty here is that every mother, every pregnancy and every baby are different: what is right for one may not be right for another.' Midwife, Sophie Adams (@mythbusting_midwife)

USING THE BRAIN

~~~

There's a popular acronym (often used in hypnobirthing, see page 182) called the BRAIN tool that can be used any time you need to make a decision or are being given a recommendation. It stands for:

Benefit – what are the benefits of this option?

Risk – what are the risks of this option?

Alternative – is there an alternative that might be more suitable for you?

Instinct – your maternal instinct can be strong at times and usually very helpful.

Nothing – what happens if you do nothing? You might not always have to act (unless it's an emergency). Can you wait and see?

Sometimes women say things like: 'I wasn't allowed' or 'they took me for a C-section'. If you take away anything from this section, take this:

No one can do anything to you without your full, informed consent.

Doctors and midwives are there to talk you through and explain options based on evidence, but you're in control. UK law protects all women during birth, nothing can be done *to you* without informed consent (the very rare exception is if a woman lacks mental capacity, and I have only experienced this twice in ten years).

'If you don't know your options, you don't have any.'

— DIANNA KORTE, BIRTH DOULA

Having talked about choice, it is important that we get the balance right. Midwives and doctors have a responsibility to protect and promote health and wellbeing throughout pregnancy, labour, birth and the postnatal period. Putting the physical and psychological safety of the people in their care first involves a lot of complex considerations and you won't be recommended to have medical intervention for absolutely no reason. There *will* be a reason, but to ensure that is the *right* reason for you personally, you may just need to ask a few more questions using the BRAIN tool.

I have seen comments on social media and forums from non-professionals telling women things like 'do not accept medical intervention' or 'you do not need *any* drugs, natural is best.' Always remember that it is never that black and white. But more importantly, it is impossible for anyone to give you accurate advice who does not have a qualification in maternity healthcare, obstetrics or midwifery, and does not know your medical history, current condition, health and personal circumstances fully. Even if the advice comes from well-meaning friends, relatives or online influencers, they need to have the right qualifications and experience and to fully understand what has led up to your current situation.

Sometimes people go on their own personal experience, what they have heard or seen, and don't necessarily understand the physiological implications or the risks involved when giving out advice. The classic comparison of one personal experience like 'my nan smoked a pack of cigarettes a day and lived to 95' are out-of-the-ordinary cases. This tells us absolutely nothing about average experiences. Smoking may not cause lung cancer in every person who smokes, but that doesn't mean to say it doesn't significantly increase the average risk. Be mindful of who and how you accept advice into your own decision-making.

What do your results mean?

If any intervention is recommended or a routine test comes back as 'abnormal' it can be hard to really translate what that risk or abnormal result means. For example, if I told you that a condition you have is 'common' can you accurately picture what that looks like in real terms? The RCOG's (Royal College of Obstetrics and Gynaecology) have a table of the phrases used to describe risk by healthcare professionals. This is helpful to see so you can get a more accurate picture of probability:

Very common: 1 in 1 to 1 in 10 = A person in family

Common: 1 in 10 to 1 in 100 = A person in street

Uncommon: 1 in 100 to 1 in 1000 = A person in village

Rare: 1 in 1000 to 1 in 10,000 = A person in small town

Very rare: Less than 1 in 10,000 = A person in large town

How you interpret these figures is individual to you and comes down to your upbringing, life experiences and your personal attitude to risk. For example, I can explain the evidence based on the risk of going more than 41+5 days overdue and the risk of induction to two different women. One woman would want an induction ASAP and another woman would think induction was unnecessary and choose further monitoring instead.

How you *feel* about your decision is important because you don't want to have a passive role in the decisions surrounding your pregnancy and birth. It is normal to feel nervous about your pregnancy and the decisions you make, but overall you want to feel calm, confident and in control as much as possible. That is how your midwives and doctors should make you feel.

KEY POINTS

- Your situation is unique so there's no one blueprint to follow for pregnancy and motherhood.
- Remember to use the BRAIN tool when presented with decision-making.
- Everyone perceives risk differently.
- Midwives and doctors are there to help you, not take over.
- Ask as many questions as you need to.
- Informed consent is a legal requirement.
- Midwives, doctors and hospitals have a duty of care and don't advise intervention without a reason but that doesn't mean you have to have it.
- Find out what will be covered at each appointment and tell us what you need in advance, if possible.
- You always have choices: you're a parent not a patient.

Modern midwifery

MIDWIFERY GETS A lot of media coverage at the moment due to TV programmes such as *Call The Midwife* or *One Born Every Minute*, but many people don't know what we are actually trained to do and how your midwife can really help you. Pregnancy and birth are often sensationalised for TV drama. A study conducted on *One Born Every Minute* found that there were no home births televised and the range of births in a midwifery-led unit were not presented clearly. This could potentially lead viewers to the impression that it is normal to give birth with medical intervention, on a labour ward with doctors in or around the birth room. This is not an accurate reflection of birth for many women and it isn't a true representation of midwifery either. I could go on about the media's version of birth, but you get the idea – it's more for entertainment and less about birth education.

What you really need to know is that midwives are your best allies throughout pregnancy, birth and the postnatal weeks. Your midwife knows the emotional and physical ins-and-outs of what you are going through; they know that no two women are the same. Even if you do see different midwives (which is now becoming less common) midwives have a range of experience and can help *you*. In this section you're going find out about what midwives *really* do behind the scenes, the future of midwifery and what that means for you, and how you can make the most out of our particular skill set.

WE ARE TRAINED PROFESSIONALS

You have to be really dedicated to midwifery and truly care for women and their babies in order to graduate. It is a lot of hard work! There is a phenomenal amount to learn. As a student, understanding medical terminology felt like learning another language. It's not just the names of conditions and the abbreviations used, the names of drugs and antibiotics are so long and hard to say let alone spell … 'Amoxa-what?'

You are tested on both your theory and practical skills. There's a test towards the end of the course called the OSCE (Objective Structured Clinical Examination); you're taken into a skills laboratory with about three examiners and are introduced to a scenario that goes something like: This is Mary, she's had a vaginal birth and lost 500ml of blood, off you go. You then need to improvise and physically show the examiners what you would do and talk them through all your decision-making providing explanation and rationale. That's just one exam. There are about 18 in total.

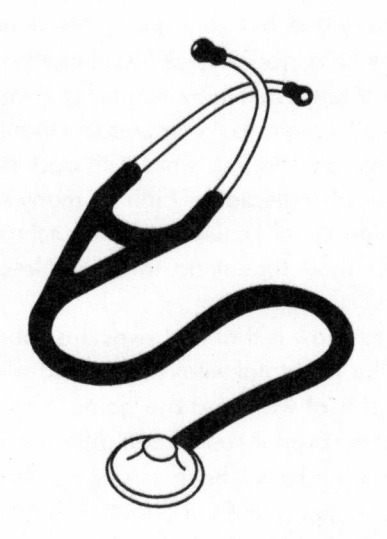

Testing continues after you've qualified too; you then need to complete your preceptorship (a period to guide and support all newly qualified midwives to make the transition from student and to develop their practice further) and demonstrate a wide variety of other skills under supervision by senior colleagues. Your skills are observed and signed off once you have proven you are competent, and the senior colleague who signs you off is accountable for doing so.

After passing your midwifery degree and completing your preceptorship you still need to update your skills regularly. We have continuing professional development (CPD), revalidation with the Nursing and Midwifery Council (NMC) and mandatory training to ensure we are up to date with the latest research and guidelines. If you don't complete your professional duties, you can't work as a midwife. It's that simple.

We are experts in natural pregnancy and birth but are trained to recognise when things are starting to deviate from the norm. You never, ever, stop learning or think you know it all in midwifery. Science and policies adjust their position based on the latest research and findings and as a qualified midwife you need to be doing that too.

The NMC are one of the world's biggest professional regulators and to practise midwifery in the UK you need to be registered with them. They work to ensure that nurses, midwives and nursing associates have the knowledge and skills to deliver consistent, quality care that keeps people safe. Their future midwife standards are being revised and as part of their five-year plan for improvement the NMC have also released 'Shaping the future themes.' Candace Imison, Director of Strategy Development at the NMC, said:

'We really wanted to make a difference in the way we developed our new strategy that will take us from 2020 to 2025. Crucially, it's the "how" we went about doing it that is almost as important as what we want to see at the final end point.

'The "how" has absolutely been about working in partnership to coproduce our strategic aims with those professionals on our register, with our partners, with the public and with our colleagues within the NMC as well.

'By developing our future work in an inclusive way, we can be much better placed in ensuring this meets the needs of professions, aligns with the work of our partners, meets the expectations that the public has – and ultimately – will help the NMC to do the best job that we possibly can for the benefit of everyone who wants to experience better, safer nursing and midwifery care.'

If you would like to take part in shaping the future of nursing and midwifery based on your experiences, head to www.nmc.org.uk/about-us/shaping-the-future to find out more.

It's important for you to know all this about modern midwifery, because you need to be able to *trust* your midwife and make use of her skills.

SUPPORTING YOUR FEMALE PHYSIOLOGY

Midwives are experts in normal, natural pregnancy and birth. We appreciate and know how to support your natural female physiology and things like the precious flow of natural oxytocin during birth – the main hormone responsible for labour progression and bonding. We understand and see the physiology of pregnancy, birth and breastfeeding working perfectly well, time after time. Midwives trust and understand these processes and can help you have the best chance of having a normal pregnancy, natural birth and smoother postnatal period.

Doctors are brilliant at dealing with complications and high-risk pregnancies as their expertise lies with abnormalities and medical treatment. I have referred women to doctors and have been so grateful for their help because they have a different set of skills to midwives. One element that makes midwifery safe in the UK is access to good medical back-up should you need it. Doctors do not need to deal with low-risk pregnancies nor do they attend home births or observe birth in the way that midwives do. Doctors sometimes see things differently to us because they specialise in situations where a woman becomes unwell or something is abnormal. Midwives see both normal and abnormal, so we have an aerial perspective. We recognise when things are progressing normally and hang back, and we intervene if this changes or refer on; making sure we always stand by a woman and her decision so that we are a true advocate for her.

WE ARE THERE FOR YOU

One of our skills is reserving judgement and simply speaking the truth; you can talk to midwives like you are talking to a friend. Sometimes women are a little nervous or not sure if they can 'say that'. Please say whatever you want, however you want. No question is a silly question. If something is bothering you, whether that is physical symptoms or feelings of anxiousness, your midwife has probably heard it before. Talk about whatever is on your mind.

Whether you see a midwife at home, at a clinic or in a hospital, we know that you are at the centre of your own care – midwives will follow *your* lead. Our primary focus is hearing about what you want so we can then give you the best care possible.

Midwives work holistically, so we're good at digging deeper to get to know your personal circumstances, especially if you have a problem. We look at the root cause of the problem, not just the treatment. The finer details about you matter because it means we can fully support you in whatever situation you are in. Sometimes I have suspected that patients are bending the truth, but I can promise you that there is no reason to. First, I am bound to confidentiality, and secondly, we tend to work it out! **We are always on your side** and want to help you, so even you feel like it's embarrassing, sounds silly or you don't think it's possible to achieve, being honest really helps us work as a team. Your midwife can only be your best advocate once you have that open level of honesty.

We are here for you, no matter what. Whether you have a vaginal birth or a C-section, bottle-feed or breastfeed, we are on your side. Whether you are 18 or 45, speak English, Russian or Swahili, are single or have six other children with your childhood sweetheart – we are right behind you. Midwives are autonomous professionals that are up-to-date with evidence-based information so if you want to run something by us or check something out we can be a good source of information, know specific resources to signpost you to and support you. Just tell us what you need and we will do our best to help you achieve it. Having this transparency between midwife and mother is so important.

CONTINUITY OF CARER

~~~

There are plans in the NHS to provide most women with continuity of carer by March 2021; this is where a woman sees the same midwife who is responsible for her care throughout pregnancy birth and postnatally.

It is being recognised by leading health organisations and authorities that midwifery-led care leads to better outcomes, less intervention and more positive memories of birth. A 2016 review on the Cochrane database (it includes over 17,000 mothers and babies at time of publication) suggests that women who received midwife-led care were less likely to experience intervention and were more likely to be satisfied with their care. The Better Births Campaign (which you should look into further if you get the chance) highlights how midwifery-led approach ensures women are at the centre of their own care.

I recently had the opportunity to shadow some of the most senior midwives in England, Claire Mathews and Jaqueline Dunkley-Bent. Their persistence, vision and dedication to make England one of the safest places on earth to give birth is remarkable. Their aim is for most women to have access to continuity of carer by 2021 and they are working tirelessly to achieve this. The momentum of change across England towards achieving this is fantastic to see: in 2018 just 2 per cent of women had continuity of carer and by March 2019, this had risen to 17.3 per cent. Some local maternity systems are already achieving over 34 per cent continuity of carer and one trust even achieved 43 per cent. The trajectory for March 2020 is 35 per cent across England and the NHS is well on its way to achieving this goal.

I have met a lot of doctors, professors and managers in my time as a midwife, but the senior midwives are more than their titles; they are midwifery pioneers. The Maternity Transformations Programme has the latest information and a useful animation that simply explains what this means for you as a pregnant woman in England, check out www.england.nhs.uk/mat-transformation for more information.

If the NHS continuity of carer model is not available in your area yet, or you live outside of England, there is another option for you, such as an independent midwife (IM). Independent midwives vary in price depending on the region. If you are interested, have a look on IMUK – it's a trusted site representing independent midwives. It is important to ensure that if you do hire an IM they are registered with the NMC and can legally look after you. If cost is a worry, many offer payment plans and may consider an exchange of skills in place of payment. Here, Louise, an IM, tells us one story:

'I recently looked after a woman whose other half can build things, so he's building me a shed rather than paying money. They are only paying for the insurance costs and are paying that in small affordable instalments. I like exchanging skills and going back to how we used to barter for services and goods! It's a myth that IMs only look after the wealthy. They are usually willing to talk openly about money and how they can help families afford their care.'

Lou Pouget, Independent Midwife

Whatever care you chose to have – NHS, private or independent midwifery care – feeling safe is the most important thing. If you feel well-supported and respected then you will have a better overall experience.

If you are having any issues with your midwife or care provider, then you need to address them ASAP. If you are under NHS care, the line manager, head of midwifery or the patient liaison service (Patient Advice and Liaison Service (PALS)) can help you to address your concerns. You aren't being a diva by doing this; disagreements or disconnection can lead to tension so it's better to get it resolved. You need to feel calm, confident and in control throughout your pregnancy and birth.

Always remember that you may not be a maternity expert but you are an expert in *your* body and you know your preferences. That is why it is important to partner with a professional that you trust to help make decisions in line with your vision and values. They will understand how you personally perceive risk and what you would like. Whether that is an epidural as early as possible or a drug-free birth behind your garden tree, we are here for you.

'Modern midwifery is about promoting a holistic, woman-centred, social model of care. This model takes into consideration the biological, psychological and social aspects of pregnancy and birth. It is important for new parents to balance evidenced-based information with their intuition and really think about what is right for them in their individual circumstances. All women deserve to be central in decision-making and feel supported in their choices by their care providers.'

Cheryl Samuels, NHS Midwife, Instagram @the_holistic_midwife, Team member @bloodtobaby

CHANGING TIMES

～～～

There has never been a time like this in human history where we have had the combination of modern medicine, ancient midwives' wisdom, technology and access to so much information at our fingertips. All generations of midwives, doctors and scientists that have gone before have allowed us to live in this unique time for women's health care.

Midwifery is one of the oldest jobs in human history and exists in virtually every human society that has ever been studied. At some points in history, midwifery has been misunderstood and was even associated with witchcraft in the fifteenth and sixteenth centuries. We've come a very long way since then and modern midwifery is stronger than ever in the UK. Elizabeth Iro, WHO's Chief Nursing Officer, celebrated International Day of the Midwife (5 May 2019) with a video referring to midwives as 'defenders of women's rights' and highlighted how we protect and promote the rights of women globally.

Midwives and doctors are bridging the gaps between traditional understanding of birth and advancement in medicine. There is a growing collaboration between mothers, midwives and obstetricians; we all respect and understand each other's roles:

You are the ultimate decision maker and the reason we are here.

Midwives support natural female physiology and recognise deviations from the norm.

Obstetricians help diagnose deviations from the norm and provide treatment for complications.

When we all work together the outcome offers women the best care humanity has ever seen.

Modern midwifery is about holding a safe space for women to allow and encourage the natural workings of their body; it is about supporting women to have access to advances in medicine and pain relief but to decline intervention when they simply don't want it. It is about making the best use of medical care when it is required. Most recently, it is about letting go of the 'natural vs medical' debate and simply working together as a team.

Modern midwifery is right at the heart of an era of change for women and I couldn't be prouder of the progress we have made.

KEY POINTS

- Midwives are safe, expert guardians of normality but support modern advancements in medical management of pregnancy and birth.
- Your midwife is right beside you, no question is a silly question.
- Make the most of your appointments and tell your midwife if you need more support.
- We are all on the same team, aiming at the same goal; there's no 'us' and 'them'.
- Letting go of 'natural vs medical' is part of modern midwifery.

Food and fuel for life

IN THIS PART we will cover what is best to eat during pregnancy and how to have a healthier pregnancy. I have asked Laura Hughes, my friend and expert in pre- and postnatal nutrition from The Pregnancy Food Company, to help me cover the most important things you need to know about food, and she's got some easy, yummy recipes for you too, later in this section.

I am pretty sure you'll agree that food to avoid in pregnancy is generally well covered these days and you will be given a list by your midwife at your booking appointment. You can also get decent and reliable advice from www.nhs.uk/conditions/pregnancy-and-baby/foods-to-avoid-pregnant.

But when it comes to making choices about what to actually put *into* your body, things can get confusing and different people say different things. You may be fortunate enough to be approached by total strangers, colleagues and others and receive random dietary advice. It usually goes something like: 'I see you've got a tuna sandwich; did you know that you can't eat tuna when you're pregnant?' I have heard some weird and wonderful 'advice' that women have been given. Some people suddenly take on a public health role around pregnant women and just can't help projecting their opinion onto you. As long as you're in the know, it is usually best to smile and nod. And for the record, you *can* eat tuna in pregnancy; you just need to limit your intake due to mercury levels. Two cans a week is plenty for most, but the official guidelines state that you can have up to four.

FACTS ABOUT FOOD

Your diet and nutrition during pregnancy can affect your baby's development and long-term health, which we will cover in a moment. Although jumping into this this may be a bit heavy for some, it is worth knowing about the relationship you are creating with your baby through food.

There's a sad but valuable study that has taught us just how much of an impact food intake has on a growing baby in the womb; the Dutch Hunger Winter Study. In the winter and spring of 1944 the German occupation limited rations to everyone, including around 40,000 pregnant women; the famine affected people of all social classes. In the Netherlands and Amsterdam people received as little as 400–800 calories per day. By 1945 the hunger was over and access to food returned to normal.

The Dutch Hunger Winter study was published 32 years later, having looked into the long-term effects of this food deprivation. It provides one of the only human experiments on the effects of intrauterine (pregnancy) deprivation on adult health.

The people who were born to pregnant women during this time were generally more obese, had more incidence of diabetes, heart disease and higher blood pressure later on in life. The intrauterine experience of hunger seems to have changed their body for life. These babies grew and developed whilst experiencing scarcity, but were then born into a world of abundance and their bodies struggled to adapt.

What we can take from this rare study is the fact that what you eat tells your baby a kind of story about the world they coming into and that they use this information to adapt their body during pregnancy to prepare for the outside world. So what you eat during pregnancy does matter, but don't worry; there are lots of simple things you can do to help you and your baby be as healthy as possible.

WHAT'S BEST TO EAT DURING PREGNANCY?

~~~~

Laura Hughes, owner of The Pregnancy Food Company hopes to help women all over the world have happier, healthier pregnancies. Here are her top tips and recipe recommendations:

It's not always easy to eat a balanced diet during pregnancy; cravings, morning sickness and tiredness all contribute to different, perhaps less than ideal, food choices. However, our requirement for micronutrients increases during pregnancy, so combining a wide variety of good-quality protein, fat and carbohydrates will help provide these essential micronutrients. And as we have just learnt, our diet does have an effect on the baby we are growing inside our tummies! Whilst we don't need to stress or obsess over having the 'perfect' diet, we certainly do need to be mindful of what we are putting in our bodies.

- Take a pregnancy or breastfeeding multivitamin **supplement** throughout pregnancy and for at least six months after birth or for the duration of breastfeeding. Do not take supplements containing vitamin A in retinol form, as too much could harm your baby. Always check the label. There are now a whole range of 'food-grown' supplements on the market that are absorbed better by the body as they contain nutrients in their natural form.
- Take an algae-based omega-3 and vitamin D3 supplement.
- The NHS recommends 400mcg per day of folic acid from when you try to conceive to the first 12 weeks of pregnancy. The best version of folic acid is the natural form 'methylfolate' or 'folate'.
- It is also now widely recommended that a daily 10mcg supplement of Vitamin D3 is taken every day in the winter in the UK, and in the summer too if you don't get much direct sunlight.
- Try to eat **protein** with every meal. Protein consists of amino acids, which are literally the 'building blocks of life'; very useful when growing a new human! Eating protein with each meal also helps to control blood sugar levels, which are often harder to control as the placenta releases hormones interrupting our insulin response. Protein can come in many forms, some of which include: chickpeas, lentils, lean meats, fish, free-range eggs and peas.
- **Carbohydrates** provide essential energy for the body (much needed in pregnancy and post-partum!) and are also a great source of fibre, vitamins, minerals and antioxidants. Try to source your carbohydrates from vegetables, whole fruits and wholegrains. It's a good idea to pair your carbohydrates with some fat or protein rather than having them 'naked' to prevent blood sugar spikes. Ideally, we would be eating up to eight portions of veg and two portions of fruit each and every day. Good

sources of carbohydrate include vegetables, wholegrain bread, pasta, rice and oats. If you are dealing with nausea and food aversions, don't worry! It's both normal and okay to eat more carbs during this phase – it can help ease the nausea. If you do only feel like eating toast or similar, try to pair it with a fat or protein, such as nut butter, to slow the absorption of sugars.

- Include **healthy fats** every day: olive oil, avocado, nuts, seeds, small oily fish (see page 55) and butter. Fats are essential for hormone production, skin elasticity, brain development, absorption of fat-soluble vitamins and many other functions in the body. If you consume dairy, buy the full-fat kind rather than the zero-fat – full-fat is packed full of vitamins, probiotics and calcium. Man-made 'trans fats' found in shop-bought cookies, cakes and in margarine should be avoided.

- **Hydrate**! Adequate water assists the stretching of the skin as your belly grows, the increase in blood volume and amniotic fluid, and also helps reduce the frequency of headaches and tiredness. Aim for two litres a day.

A WORD ON ORGANIC

I recommend you buy organic produce where you can. Not all of us can afford organic all the time though so look up the 'Clean 15 and Dirty Dozen' list (www.ewg.org/foodnews/clean-fifteen.php) to find out how you can avoid the foods with the most chemicals.

Unfortunately, a lot of the time the healthier, most nutritious foods are the more expensive options. If you are in need of financial support you may well be eligible for the Healthy Start scheme. This is a means-tested scheme that gives you vouchers to spend with local retailers. Pregnant women and children over one and under four years old are eligible. Healthy Start also provides a vitamins scheme especially for pregnant and breastfeeding women. Check out www.healthystart.nhs.uk/healthy-start-vouchers/do-i-qualify to see if you are eligible. Do look at frozen and canned veg too which can be more affordable, and just as nutritious (frozen, especially). You can even get frozen avocado and edamame beans.

VEGETARIAN AND VEGAN DIETS

These can be successfully maintained throughout pregnancy and breastfeeding with a bit of careful planning. Make sure to include the following, and speak to your midwife or a nutritionist about your specific needs too.

- Nutritional yeast for extra B12 should be included daily – fortified Engevita yeast flakes are a good source to try.
- Iron-rich foods such as dark leafy greens and lentils should be eaten with a source of vitamin C, such as peppers or tomatoes, to improve absorption.
- Vitamin D from free-range egg yolks (which also provide choline), the sun or a supplement.
- Buckwheat, hemp and quinoa for sources of complete protein.
- Nuts, seeds and dark leafy greens for sources of iron and zinc.
- Seaweed for a good source of iodine and iron.
- Sesame seeds, broccoli, cabbage, tahini and pulses for calcium.
- Soaked wholegrains, beans and legumes.
- It is essential to include a high quality pregnancy supplement every day as we cannot obtain everything we need from food sources.

LOOKING AFTER YOURSELF

You have a lot on at the moment, but eating well will help support you during this busy time. Here are a few ideas that my clients have found useful to help them eat well:

- Follow the 80/20 system; with 80 per cent of your foods being as healthy as possible and being more relaxed about the other 20 per cent. This can help to make eating healthily more relaxed and positive; you don't have to eat 'perfectly' all the time.
- Cooking from scratch is ideal so we know what is going into our foods. Batch-cooking can be a lifesaver here. Take it one meal at a time if you

aren't used to cooking much or you might want to look into the delivery box schemes that provide you with ingredients to cook from scratch.

- Snacks can pack in the nutrients. Try and plan ahead with your snacks so you don't have to grab a muffin or whatever when out and about. Apples and nut butter, carrot sticks and hummus, nuts and berries and boiled eggs are great snack choices, as they all contain protein.
- Get yourself a good-quality water bottle to carry around with you – a glass one is ideal. If using a plastic bottle you already own, check that it is BPA-free (Bisphenol-A has links with endocrine disruption).
- Green smoothies can be very helpful if you are struggling to get nutrients in. You can even make one up and freeze it into suckable ice cubes if that helps with nausea.
- Avoid artificial sweeteners and processed foods as much as possible. As a general rule, if you can't pronounce the ingredient, it shouldn't be eaten!
- Try to eat seasonally. A list of seasonal produce is easily found online and can really help boost nutrient value, as well as give you more variety.
- Aim to eat salmon, mackerel or sardines at least twice a week. Tuna (canned or fresh) can be enjoyed too, but two cans a week is ample. Avoid bigger fish, such as swordfish and marlin, as they contain high levels of mercury.
- Soft cheeses can be eaten as long they are pasteurised (many are) or cooked, such as baked camembert.
- Salad, veg and fruit should always be washed well with clean water.
- Meat or shellfish should be well cooked.
- Smoked salmon and sushi is OK to enjoy providing it has been frozen and defrosted to kill off bacteria and parasites. Most supermarket smoked salmon will have been frozen first – check the packet to be sure.
- Sugary drinks and foods really do need to be limited due to the effect on baby's metabolic health, and your own blood sugar levels. 'Diet' drinks with sweeteners aren't great either as they can contain unhealthy additives.
- Nuts are safe to eat in pregnancy and are a good source of protein – as long as you aren't allergic, of course.
- If you have very old non-stick pans, you might like to swap your cooking pots and pans to cast iron or stainless steel, as old pans can release nasty chemicals when heated.

PREGNANCY SUPER RECIPES

If you are struggling for inspiration in your cooking, why not try some of these recipes. They are all packed with nutrition so you will feel you are really looking after yourself.

CHEWY GINGER AND APRICOT BISCUITS

These are great for morning sickness. Ginger has been used for centuries as an antiemetic (anti-sickness). The chewy apricots, molasses and egg yolks are ideal for providing a boost to vitamins and minerals you may be missing when experiencing morning sickness. If you'd prefer to make vegan versions of these biscuits, just swap the butter for coconut oil (make sure you add a pinch of salt to the recipe too), and the egg yolks can be replaced with a flax egg.

MAKES 24

200g rye flour
3 level tsp ground ginger
1 heaped tsp cinnamon

60g dried apricots
60g salted butter
60g blackstrap molasses
2 egg yolks

Measure out the rye flour into a mixing bowl, then add the ginger and cinnamon and mix thoroughly.

Cut the dried apricots into small little chunks, about the size of a raisin. Alternatively, you could whizz in a blender. Add these to the rye flour mix.

Next, measure out the butter and molasses into a saucepan, put on a low heat and stir until the mixture is melted and is warmed through (alternatively, you can use the microwave; just pop it on defrost and do 30-second blasts until melted).

Add the butter mixture to the flour and mix well. Add the egg yolks and mix again.

Cover the mixing bowl and place in the fridge for 20 minutes.

Meanwhile, heat the oven to 175°C/350°F and take the mixing bowl out of the fridge. Divide the mixture into 24 balls, rolling with your hands. If you find the mixture sticky to handle, dust your hands with a little rye flour.

Line a baking sheet with baking paper and place the balls, equally spaced – you might need two trays – with 12 biscuits on each. Now push down on each ball with the palm of your hand to squash down into a nice biscuit shape. Bake in the oven for 12 minutes. Cool on a wire rack.

Once cooled you can eat them straight away, or they will keep in an airtight container for five days or in the freezer for three months.

BANANA AND CASHEW CHIA 'PORRIDGE'

During pregnancy it's really important to get a source of protein in at every meal. This recipe packs in the protein to keep you feeling fuller for longer – growing a baby is hungry work! It also helps to keep your blood sugar level more stable which is essential during pregnancy. Banana contains potassium and vitamin B6 which can help combat morning sickness. Make this the night before and leave in the fridge, or in the morning. Double-up if you like; this will last in the fridge for up to two days.

SERVES 1

100ml any nut milk
30g chia seeds
1 tbsp cashew nut butter

½ banana, sliced or mashed (you can use frozen)
1 tsp cinnamon
1 tsp vanilla extract

OPTIONAL TOPPINGS
1 tbsp frozen or fresh berries (use a mix of raspberries, blackberries, redcurrants and/or blueberries)

1 tsp black sesame seeds (regular sesame seeds are fine too)

Combine all the ingredients in a bowl or large glass. You can use a food processor if you like a smooth consistency, or just mix with a spoon.

When ready to eat, add the berries and sesame seeds.

FOOD FOR THOUGHT

Being as healthy as possible in pregnancy isn't just about what you are eating, it is also about your relationship with food and everything else you are putting into your amazing body. I know this is something the women I see think about, and it's certainly something I work on. I used to think nothing of shoving a sandwich in my face whilst rushing to work and grabbing food on the go until I learnt about mindful eating.

Mindful eating is simply being as aware as possible each time you eat; this helps change your perception of food and places more of a focus on 'what will give me and my baby the most nutrients?' That way you will naturally lean towards the healthier option. Of course, there will be days where you need to grab something quick and easy on the go; it just shouldn't be a habit.

Being mindful about what you are eating, but feeling miserable about depriving yourself, defeats the object. So, if you've got a sweet tooth and often fancy a dessert then maybe share one? That way you've had a treat but not overdone it on the sugar and you have really enjoyed each mouthful. Win-win! As already mentioned, something that seems to work for many of the women is the 80/20 rule (see page 54); it is important to enjoy treats. You deserve them too.

WEIGHT GAIN

There are no formal, evidence-based guidelines from the UK government or other professional bodies on the amount of weight women should gain in pregnancy – although it is often debated. What we do know is that heart disease and diabetes are seriously on the increase and those diagnosed are younger than ever before. The British Heart Foundation and Diabetes UK have recent and rather concerning statistics on the prevalence and serious health implications these two bring with them. I am all for being body-positive; how you feel about and talk to yourself is so important – your body is amazing! But it is also important that I am upfront and honest with you: your weight can really affect your risks during pregnancy. Managing being overweight may not be as simple as 'eat less and do more' – I understand there is a lot more to why women are increasingly overweight or obese.

Rather than focusing on weight gain, it is better to understand how to be healthier and the recommended increase in calorie intake. Most people know eating for two is not good for you; it's all over the press and in most pregnancy books. But what that means in real terms is that you don't actually need to increase your calorie intake until the third trimester – that's just from 28 weeks until the end of your pregnancy. From that point on, it is currently recommended that eating an extra 200 calories per day is sufficient for providing the extra energy you need. That looks like a handful of dried apricots; it really isn't much. The only exception to this is if you have a very active lifestyle, say working on a farm or teaching exercise classes all day; then you may need a little extra energy intake right from the start of your pregnancy.

ALCOHOL

No one really knows the safe amount pregnant women can consume, so national guidelines recommend pregnant women do not drink alcohol throughout their entire pregnancy.

Not drinking alcohol during the first trimester is definitely a good idea because this is the most crucial point of development. After that, some women tell me that they enjoy the odd glass of wine. According to the research available and several other experts, one unit once a week 'probably' won't do either of you any harm.

The fact is, we don't know enough about what even minimal alcohol consumption does in pregnancy. What we do know is that alcohol passes across the placenta, so the more you drink the more your baby receives. The evidence on drinking during pregnancy is complex because everyone has different lifestyles. A woman who has a well-balanced diet, good emotional support, does regular exercise and has the odd glass of wine *should* be fine. When a woman has other risk factors, stressors and an unhealthy lifestyle, perhaps drinking isn't a good idea.

COFFEE AND CAFFEINE INTAKE

I'm a coffee addict and I'm far from being alone here. You might not be a coffee fan, but there is caffeine in many drinks, so read on.

The bad news is that a few credible and large-scale studies have come to the same conclusion: high caffeine intake can increase the risk of miscarriage, reduce placental blood flow and therefore the flow of nutrients to your baby, which can impact growth and development.

The good news is that there is an amount of coffee you can drink safely. For those of you who don't drink coffee, you also need to factor in caffeine in fizzy drinks, chocolate and tea.

For precaution, most experts agree that up to 200mg of caffeine per day is safe. To be honest, that meant nothing to me so here is a guide:

1 mug instant coffee = 100mg   1 can of energy drink = 80mg
1 cup filter coffee = 140mg   1 dark chocolate bar (42g) = 25mg
1 can of coke = 40mg   1 milk chocolate bar (42g) = 15mg

WHAT ELSE IS GOING INTO YOUR BODY?

It might surprise you to realise that we ingest chemicals through our make-up and beauty products. We are also exposed to chemicals when out and about; car fumes, etc. Here are some tips to help you reduce your exposure to harmful chemicals, which is important at any stage of life, and especially in pregnancy.

Chemicals

Avoiding harmful chemicals is near impossible these days. Overall try to use natural beauty products and avoid conventional cleaning products in the home. A website that has a wealth of information about product safety is www. ewg.org.

Some chemicals in particular are thought to be more harmful than others during pregnancy and a few of these can easily be avoided:

Parabens: Also known as propylparaben, butylparaben, isopropy-lparaben and methylparabens. They are mostly used as preservatives in cosmetics like foundation and lipstick to prevent them from growing bacteria.

Phthalates: Most commonly found in scented products like soaps, perfumes and shampoos.

Formaldehyde: Found in things like nail polish, eyelash glue and various other products. Some studies have shown that formaldehyde exposure could cause cancer and in 2016 the chemical was classified as a carcinogen in the UK.

That isn't to say you need to chuck out all your make-up and never get nails or lashes done; it is just good to be aware of your chemical exposure during pregnancy. There are other options and more natural products on the market. You can make your own nourishing lotions from things like coconut oil, rosehip oil or shea butter too.

FRESH AIR

Your environment is really important too. Getting fresh air is really good for your health – not exactly a news flash, I know, but this can sometimes be forgotten – getting fresh air for your placenta matters. If you live or work near a busy road or in a built-up area, try and get out to a park, or out of the city, as often as possible. Getting a few house plants can help filter the air around you too (see page 72 for more on this).

If you are thinking of painting the nursery bedroom for your baby, it is important to ensure the paint is safe; try to opt for an eco-paint that is water-based, and has zero volatile organic compounds (VOCs).

Many carpets contain chemicals, especially if plastic-based; if you get a new carpet make sure it is fitted at least two months before the baby is due as the chemicals linger for a while.

Having a healthy pregnancy is all about balance. Realistically, eating a brownie or getting a take-away every now and then isn't going to put you or your baby at risk. If you eat nutritious food most of the time, try to relax, stay active, get out in the fresh air and avoid harsh chemicals as much as possible, overall you are being as healthy as you can be. In reality, it's not about the one-offs, it's about the daily things you do.

KEY POINTS

- Food really is fuel for the life you are growing.
- Your baby is developing and getting cues from your food intake – opt for nutrient-rich food as much as possible.
- Nourishing yourself is important during pregnancy, and beneficial for baby too.
- Try to eat a variety of fresh, wholesome food where possible. Aim for a good mixture of protein, vegetables, fruits, fats, and carbohydrates.
- Alcohol can pass through to the placenta during pregnancy, and the advice is to limit the amount you drink.
- Watch your caffeine intake; it can really creep up if you love coffee, tea and chocolate.
- Try the 80/20 rule to get a great balance between eating well and the occasional treat. Enjoy your food and don't be too hard on yourself.
- Consider everything you are putting into your body – get fresh air and avoid harsh chemicals.

Your baby shares your body *and* your mind

WHAT BABIES LEARN in the womb has really captivated me, for as long as I can remember. I have spent hours on my own in the library researching their secret lives. When we think about pregnancy we understandably think about the physical elements but how babies learn and develop is down to both your body and your mind. In this section we will run through what babies do in there, how you can really help your baby learn before they are born, and the importance of your emotional wellbeing. Some of what is to come may sound far-fetched at times, but when you break it down to a cellular level (the most basic structural units of the human body) it makes total sense.

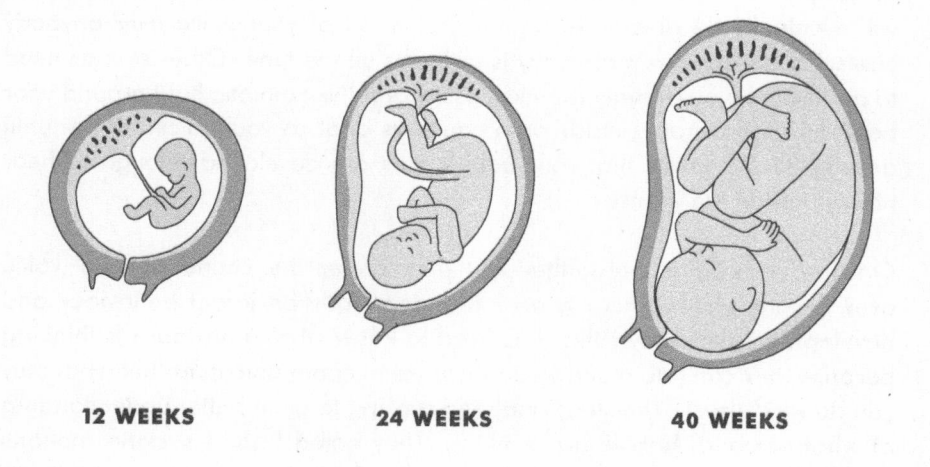

12 WEEKS   **24 WEEKS**   **40 WEEKS**

WHAT DO BABIES DO IN THE WOMB?

You and your baby are connected in so many ways, and your baby is learning what it is like to be alive through you, your body and your experiences. Some of the most important development and learning your baby will do is with you during pregnancy. Your bodies are well and truly connected through a cocktail of hormones, sounds, touch, movement and tastes. In some ways, your baby shares a little bit of everything you do, which is just one of the reasons you needed to draw that sacred circle around yourself from day one (see page 5).

During my travels around the medical library I came across an exciting field of science called the Fetal Origins Hypothesis; it concludes that when you hold your baby for the first time they already know so much about you and have already been shaped by you. Unborn babies are aware of sounds, tastes and to some extent even your mood, so you can start to teach and interact with your baby during pregnancy.

YOUR VOICE AND OTHER SOUNDS

As early as 16 weeks, your baby will start to feel the sound of your voice and will eventually be able to recognise the sound of your voice over anybody else's. This is because your baby is with you all the time. Other sounds need to go through your tummy muscles, tissue and the amniotic fluid around your baby, so sounds from outside aren't quite as clear as your voice. It's not until around 22–24 weeks that your baby's ears are developed enough to hear noises outside the womb.

Once your baby is born, they will also prefer the sound of your voice over anyone else's. There is an interesting study on infant behaviour and development that shows this. It is hard to know what a newborn is thinking because they can't do much when it comes to communicating, but what they can do well is suck. The study analysed sucking to get a better understanding of what newborn babies are thinking. They noted babies sucking motions and behaviour whilst playing different sounds. Babies tend to suck slower

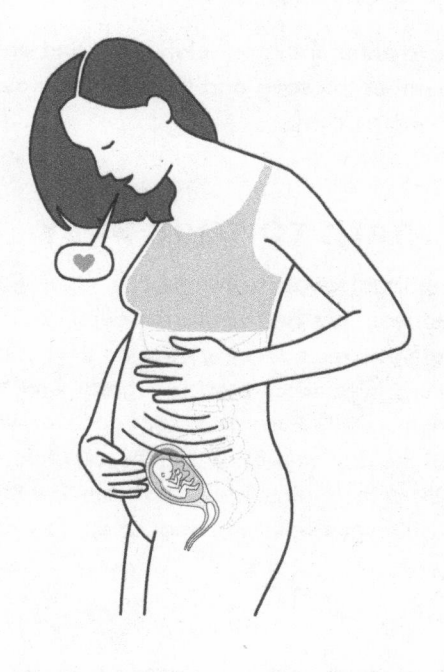

when they are interested in something, and suck quickly if they are bored. The research revealed that newborns show the most interest in their mum's voice as they generally slowed down sucking whilst they could hear mum talking.

A study by Peter Hepper in Belfast found women who watched *Neighbours* daily on TV had babies that responded to the theme tune after birth; they stopped moving, became alert and their heart rates dropped, suggesting that they actually remembered what they had heard regularly during pregnancy, and it was comforting.

Something else that really brought home just how much a baby learns in the womb is a 2010 study where researchers found that babies cry in their mum's accent. French babies cry on a raising note and German babies cry on a falling note – the different tones imitate their native language. How incredible is that? Although it may not seem like it at times, from birth your baby will be communicating specifically with you, and has even learnt how to communicate in your native language.

Play your baby music in pregnancy and relax, sway and sing – when your baby is born they will remember the song and the relaxation associated with it and this can help to calm them down.

TALK TO YOUR BABY

Your voice is so important to your growing baby. When you speak, not only can your baby hear you, but their whole spine vibrates lightly too, so they can physically feel your voice moving through them. Talking or singing to your baby during pregnancy is such a great way to start bonding. I know it may seem a silly thing to recommend as you are probably talking throughout the day anyway, but when you direct your attention to your baby and talk to them directly, it is possible that they can sense the change between what you are saying and the emotion behind it.

TEACHING YOUR BABY ABOUT FOOD

I often wondered how much babies could taste the food their mums eat in pregnancy. One of things that inspired my investigation was my dad's reaction to oranges – he hates them. So much so, you can't even peel one near him because it makes him feel sick. Oranges are probably one of my favourite fruits and it almost annoys me that he makes such a fuss about the smell. I mentioned it to my nan one day and she said, 'Funny you should say that because when I was pregnant with your dad the smell of oranges used to make me vomit, I couldn't stand them.' My dad is now 56 and showing no signs of getting closer to accepting the smell of an orange. I wanted to find out if there was a link between what my nan ate in pregnancy and my dad's preferences. Spoiler alert: there's a significant link. By the time you are 32 weeks pregnant your baby's taste buds are well developed and so are the receptors that allow them to smell. The flavours of what you eat find their way into the amniotic fluid which is swallowed by your baby.

In France, researchers found that babies born to women who ate liquorice-flavoured food and drink throughout pregnancy preferred this taste on both their first and fourth day of life. The babies born to women that didn't eat any liquorice were not impressed and made signs that translated to 'yuk!' At six months old, the babies still showed signs of preferring these tastes. Taste buds do change over time and there is some research to suggest that the memories in the womb are not carried throughout life and have limitations, so maybe your baby won't be quite as persistent about their exposures in your tummy as my dad is!

BONDING IN PREGNANCY

Finding out you are pregnant might have led to thoughts like 'Is this really a good time?' or 'Will we have the money?' or 'Oh my goodness, what are we doing?' Pregnancy is daunting and can take time to get your head around. After you have done a bit of planning and thinking, try to get a clear idea in your mind that *this* is the baby that you really want to have. Even if it takes you six months to get to this thought. This can really help you build a bond with *this* baby at *this* time in your life. Creating a bond as early as possible helps to build on your relationship; you can show your baby love before they are born. When you feel happy and excited about your baby, you release happy and relaxing hormones and your baby receives some of these hormones through your bloodstream.

In one study, researchers found that when women watched happy film clips (through ear phones so the babies couldn't hear) their babies moved more, and when they watched sad film clips, their babies moved less, potentially showing energy conservation due to stress exposure. This particular study only had ten participants, so it is far too small to prove anything conclusively, but it does hint that there could possibly be a link, and knowing what we do about the release of hormones it would make sense. Why not give it a try!

Dr Thomas R. Verny is one of the world's leading experts on the effect of the prenatal and early postnatal environment on personality development. His book *The Secret Life of the Unborn Child* is a brilliant read. He believes that everything pregnant women feel and are exposed to can, in small ways, influence the development of an unborn baby. You aren't only building a body during pregnancy, you are building a brain, another nervous system and a human who thinks.

The topic of consciousness, of when your baby's brain starts to think, is complex, well debated and not that well understood. None the less it is fascinating to understand some of the building blocks and possible timings that come into play for human development. Many experts believe consciousness isn't something that is switched on like a light, but more of a gradual turning up of the dimmer switch, but more research is needed.

At around 25 weeks, the peripheral nervous system (nerves relaying movement from the tissues and limbs outside the brain) joins up with the cerebral cortex (part of the brain that's responsible for higher thought processes like memory, attention and awareness). This is what connects the outside world to the higher brain. This doesn't mean to say that a 25-week-old baby in the womb experiences consciousness like us adults; we can't really compare our adult experience of consciousness and awareness to that of an unborn baby. It does mean that talking to your baby and bonding with this baby at this time during pregnancy is all worthwhile!

FEELING STRESSED

Many of my patients are working during their pregnancy, or are busy caring for other children. Life can be stressful, and I know this is another concern for already stressed women.

Women are under more pressure than ever to be 'successful'. We are fighting to be heard in different spaces, for the gender pay gap to be closed, for more career opportunities to be open, to feel happy in our own skin and to be seen as a good mother. Trying to do it all can lead to mums feeling anxious or perhaps overwhelmed. I want to say here: mammas, you are doing incredible things, and have nothing to prove to anyone; keep doing what *you* are doing.

Some studies have concluded that very stressed mums can have babies with a lower birth weight and even an increased risk of premature birth. However, it is important that we look at the *whole* picture here. Is the woman drinking or smoking? Is she eating well? What is causing the stress? What is her support like? Has she been a victim of discrimination or worried about finances? There is a lot more to the story than just highlighting what high levels of stress are linked to. What you define as a stressful event and what I define as a stressful event will differ, so when studied it is hard to accurately represent stress exposures. Either way, we do know that too much stress (whatever it is that you define as stressful) for long periods of time isn't good for your body, whether pregnant or not, so let's take a look at how to manage stress during your pregnancy.

The amazing thing about the human brain is that you can change how it functions. Because the parts you use most often are strengthened, practise really does make perfect. Brain-based stress management involves strengthening the wires that promote healthy coping, so the brain becomes wired to favour that pathway. The human brain loves simplicity and patterns, that's why it's so hard to kick a habit. Your brain has been reliant on that pathway for so long you need to consciously intervene and in effect rewire it. I'm not suggesting you start a load of mind-management practices now, but there are some easy things you can do to manage the normal, yet emotional, ups and downs of pregnancy and your stress levels.

The neocortex part of the brain helps to process information, and it is also one of the most modern parts of our brain. The amygdala, where we tend to process stress and aggression, is more primal. We needed that part more a few hundred years ago, but it can still become active when we are presented with something that's stressful and alarming.

What that means for us nowadays is that the body struggles to tell the difference between needing to run from a tiger or needing to meet a deadline. Through the release of hormones it puts your body in a heightened state of awareness, making you feel on edge. A lot of experts agree that babies are negatively affected by stress levels if the increase in cortisol is *often* or for *long* periods of time.

If you've had an argument with your partner or felt stressed about a work deadline, please don't worry, because some stress can even be a good lesson for unborn babies. Stress is a normal part of life and babies need some exposure to stress hormones to help learn how to manage it. There is even a link between short-term stress exposure and brain maturity. The key to keeping stress exposure on the healthy side is to ensure you *calm down* and come out of that heightened state of awareness after feeling stressed, anxious or having a disagreement.

In any stressful or difficult situation, the best thing you can do is stop and consciously re-regulate your body's stress response. You can quickly and easily do this by taking deep breaths. Breathe in deeply, hold for two seconds, and then breathe out through your mouth for four seconds. Repeat five times. If you are at work and need to calm down, go to the loo, lock the door and do your breathing exercise. No one is going to question a pregnant woman needing a wee! Even better, go out for a brisk walk and a change of scene or sit on a park bench and do some mindful breathing. Also see yogic breathing in pregnancy on page 30.

Author of *Eat Pray Love*, Elizabeth Gilbert, says, 'my hobby is writing but my job is my mental health'. I'm fascinated by her and thought that was such an interesting way of looking at our work–life balance.

During the third trimester, your baby's neurological development is at its peak, so if you are still working, or are busy looking after others, planning or decorating, make sure you take time to have a breather, to relax and let your baby know everything is okay. We can all get wrapped up in the fast pace of life, but calming your mind and your body is essential. Aim for ten minutes each day dedicated to relaxation. Literally give yourself time out. Those minutes make a difference to your mental state, leading to a change in your physiological state. Hypnobirthing is also a great way of doing this (see page 182).

If something keeps coming back to worry you then try to get out in natural surroundings. Forests, parks and longer walks have been shown to reduce the stress-related hormone cortisol by up to 12 per cent. Within five minutes your body and brain start to change, your heart rate slows, your facial muscles relax and the neocortex quietens down (that internal chatter we all have). Florence Williams, author of *The Nature Fix: Why Nature Makes Us Happier,*

Healthier and More Creative, looks at how nature impacts human health on various levels. She found the smell of pine trees can actually strengthen the immune system. If you spend an hour and a half walking around nature with live plants and animals your personal problems no longer take centre-stage and you begin to feel more connected to the people and world around you. Finnish researchers found being in nature for five hours alone can make you happier. In Japan, *shinrin-yoku* (forest-bathing) has been part of the national health programme since 1982 and is supported as a treatment by well-respected doctors.

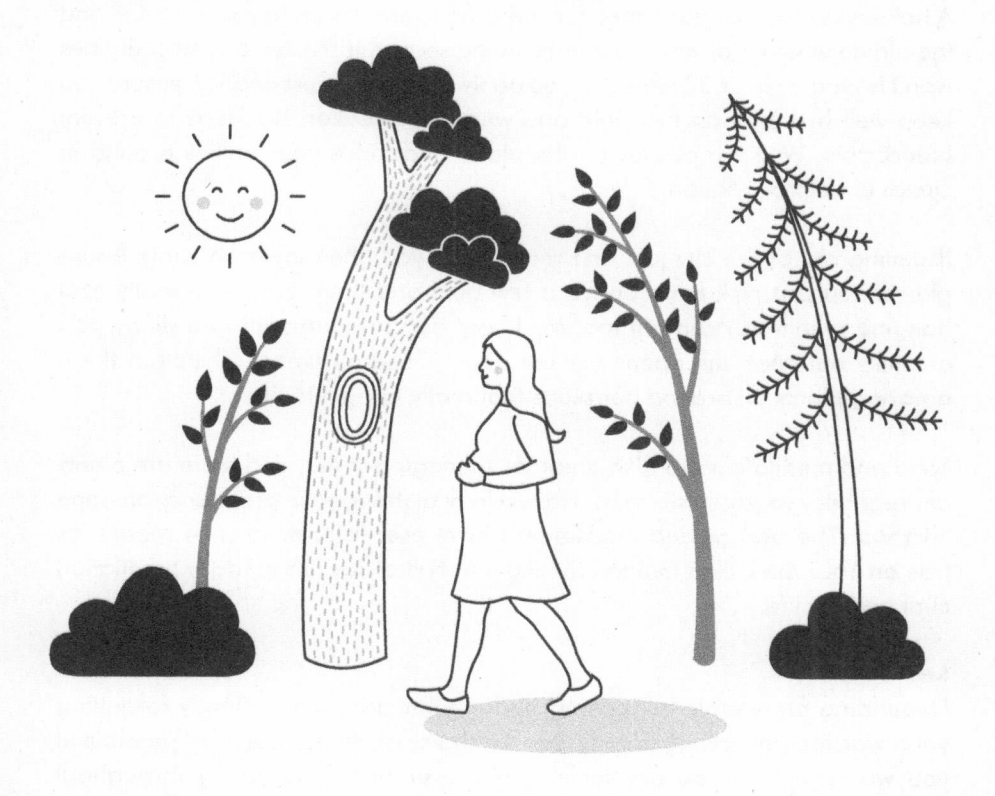

I live in London and Cornwall, and when I step off the train at either end, I can physically feel the change in atmosphere. In some cities it is almost like everyone has been given the challenge of looking like they are busiest, and their destination is the most important. Sometimes I find myself putting on a serious face to scroll through my Pinterest boards just to fit in!

If you live in a city or built-up town have a weekend away, out of the city, and visit the countryside or sea. Physically being in open space can help give you some mental space too. Until you get out, you don't realise how claustrophobic cities can be.

A holiday is always a good idea for reducing stress. It's up to you, your GP and the airline whether or not you can fly in the second trimester, but most airlines won't let you fly after 37 weeks. If you do fly during your pregnancy, ensure you keep well hydrated on the flight and wear compression stockings to prevent blood clots. Walk up and down the plane and move your ankles around in circles to help circulation.

If getting out of the city just isn't realistic for you, then invest in some house plants. You can pick them up for a few quid and there are some really cool hanging plants you can get too. My friend got an apartment in a dingy part of a city but once she opens her flat door, it doesn't matter. She's got these amazing plants all around her place that really bring it to life.

Yoga and meditation are also great for managing stress, and there are plenty of pregnancy yoga classes to try. Have a look at the yoga in pregnancy on page 115 too. The best guided meditation I have ever listened to is by Mooji; it's free on YouTube called Guided Meditation: Full of Joy. Short, daily meditation changed my life.

Let it go
Depending on what is happening during your pregnancy, simply forgetting your worries and being happy can be hard at times, but it is possible if you work on how you are feeling. Not everyone feels happy throughout their pregnancy and that's okay – as long as the *majority* of the time you are feeling content with how things are going, it's okay to feel nervous or worried. You're on a journey you've never trodden before, even if this is your second or third baby, it is a different baby, time, and therefore experience so a bit of nervousness goes with the territory. I don't want to normalise anxiety

because anxiety can be crippling but, in all honesty, a certain amount of anxiety can be normal.

Accepting and dealing with your personal circumstances may be difficult, especially if things are not turning out the way you expected. Even if they are, worrying about losing your identity, a changing relationship with your partner, how having a baby will impact your career, missing your old life, not being able to cope or what could happen is common – especially with first-time mums. The 'what if . . .' can start to go on repeat in your mind.

There's a well-known acronym that describes fear:

F – False

E – Evidence

A – Appearing

R – Real

It explains why much of what we 'fear' isn't always real or may never happen. If this is the case, accept your fear for what it is, and then try to let it go. It is easy to dwell on the things that might go wrong during pregnancy or birth, but it doesn't actually help you, and you spend all that time worrying about something that might never happen. Learning to let go of things now is not only a brilliant tool to have in your locker – and probably why all adults could relate to *Frozen's* song 'Let it Go' – but it is useful for parenthood too.

GET SOME EXERCISE

Another way to help manage stress and clear your mind is exercise. From getting your blood pumping to helping you focus on something else, exercise can help keep a handle on the hormonal ups and downs of pregnancy. Louise Gabbitas, the midwife that got to the 2019 final of Channel 4's *SAS Who Dares Wins*, has got some serious strength, but interestingly, she doesn't just focus on the physical benefits of exercise. They are kind of secondary to why she trains.

HERE ARE SOME IDEAS TO HELP YOU 'LET IT GO'

Feeling like you have too much to handle right now? Here are some ideas to help you lighten the mental load.

- Cut down on the stuff that stresses you out or doesn't make you feel good. This sounds obvious, but it may not be when you're in and amongst it. Feel free to say no to going to that event or the extra bit of work you 'should' do. *Stay in your sacred circle*; it's okay to say no to people who want things from you. Unless you have a formal contract, you're not responsible for anyone else's happiness or obliged to fulfil their wishes if you don't want to do. Even if you have a formal agreement, everything is negotiable to a certain extent. Cut the unnecessary crap down or out of your life – we've all got it – but pregnancy is a time to say 'Nah. Not today'. You've got enough on your plate and having any unnecessary extras can add to your feeling of nervousness.
- If there's stuff you normally do but are struggling to manage, ask for help and offload things. There is no shame in doing this, even if that's with the simplest of things. Also, communicate with your partner or friends about how you are feeling. It makes a huge difference and you might not need to ask for help as it may then be offered.
- Talk about how you are feeling to anyone you trust. Sometimes simply talking to someone puts things into perspective, minimises your worries and gets them out of your head into the open. Offloading helps you to process your emotions and thoughts properly.
- Start a daily gratitude log; this has been proven to reduce symptoms of depression. Think about every tiny thing you are grateful for every day. At first just take 30 seconds to think of three things you're grateful for and jot them down. Like your warm comfy bed, your nourishing breakfast, access to running water, your friends, family and anyone in your life who you love.

The basic things you may have but not everyone in the world does; welcome and remember all the positive and amazing things you have in your life. Then, if you want, build up to more personal things, like your ability to see things more clearly and get excited for your baby's birth, then add those in too. Have a quick daily thank you, or a longer, more thought-out list.

- After a stressful event or day at work, it is important to 'down regulate'. First, acknowledge that it was stressful and upsetting, let the emotion out and then down regulate using the breathing technique on page 70.

When astronauts talk about their experience of looking down at Earth, they say it is liberating. Seeing Earth from a distance makes them realise how small their own problems are. My friend is a psychologist and if I get overwhelmed, she often reminds me: 'We're all bacteria on a rock ... to the Universe, anyway.'

She works nights, does CrossFit competitions and still finds time to train daily. I thought she made some really brave and bold moves on SAS (for any of you who didn't watch it, she chose to fight a man and threw herself off the edge of a cliff with no hesitation). I asked her what exercise does for her mental health and if she had any tips for you:

'I've always said that the goal of training or exercise is good health and fitness. Good health includes being mentally healthy too.

'Good health and fitness looks different at each stage of pregnancy and it is also different from person to person; it is important to remember that. Exercise offers a chance for you to do something positive for yourself, which has the added benefit of making you feel good. It may sound a bit selfish, but actually we have come to realise that if we don't look after our own physical and mental health then we can't give our best selves to others, which is what most mothers/mothers-to-be want to be able to do – be the best mother they can.

'Exercise during pregnancy will only be positive. It gets endorphins flowing, which produces a positive feeling in the body, making you feel better about yourself both physically and mentally. With the increasing options and variety of ways of keeping fit, the motivation could be that it is something that you genuinely enjoy doing so that it doesn't become a "thing to fit in" rather a part of your day you look forward to. Looking after yourself means so much more than "trying to keep fit". It's about giving yourself and your family the healthiest version of you so that everything becomes more enjoyable.'

If the mental aspects and release of happy hormones aren't enough to sway you, a study at Queen Mary University of London might. Researchers found that women who eat healthily and stay active in pregnancy cut their chance of needing a Caesarean section. The research looked at data from 12,500 women across 16 countries and found that women of any weight who consumed a healthy diet and did regular exercise in pregnancy reduced excessive weight gain, gestational diabetes and the risk of requiring a Caesarean section. Winning! Researchers found no strong evidence to suggest that exercise and a healthy diet had a negative effect on the baby, such as being small or large for gestational age or needing admission to a neonatal intensive care unit.

Remember, exercise doesn't have to be strenuous to be beneficial, and you should never start any strenuous exercise you have not done pre-pregnancy. If you usually work out, ensure your exercises are adapted for pregnancy and always tell a trainer or instructor that you are pregnant. Gentle swims, joining a pregnancy yoga or Pilates class or going for some brisk walks are all great ways to exercise. 'I wish I didn't go for a walk' – said no one ever.

DO YOU FEEL DEPRESSED?

Having said all that, using the above self-help tools doesn't mean you should ignore feelings of depression or developing anxieties. Some women do experience mental health problems for the first time during pregnancy, and anxiety and depression are the most common. If the balance has tipped and you no longer feel happy the majority of the time, then you need to properly address how you are feeling. It's okay to admit this to yourself, to your partner and to healthcare professionals. Opening up is the best thing you can do.

STEPS TO CLEAR YOUR MIND

Feeling fed-up? Have these ideas up your sleeve:

- Remove yourself from the stress – even if that's for five minutes in the loo.
- Down regulate (see page 75), breathe or walk.
- Get out in nature as much as possible, especially forests or open spaces.
- Meditate and or join a yoga class.
- Say no, ask for help, offload and start a gratitude log.
- Exercise.

'As a perinatal psychiatrist I work with women and their families to support their mental health through pregnancy and after birth. For almost all of us, pregnancy and early motherhood is a time where we feel our moods are changeable, often in response to being tired and adapting to becoming a new mum. However, for some women these mood changes persist and they may have episodes of depression, anxiety or obsessive thoughts. This can happen in pregnancy and in the postnatal period. I want women to know that this is common and they are not a bad mum. Please don't be afraid to speak up if you feel your mood is low all the time or you can't enjoy life. Or you may feel agitated and anxious all the time and not able to eat or sleep well. It can seem so scary but try to tell someone, a partner, your GP or health visitor or someone on a helpline like the one run by the PANDAS Foundation.

'Often talking to someone can be a huge relief; it can help you feel heard and less alone. Support and healing can come in many ways; peer support, exercise, therapy, medication or supplements. You can and will feel better. You are a good mum even if you are anxious or depressed.'

Dr Rebecca Moore, Consultant Perinatal Psychiatrist and co-founder of Make Birth Better

Sometimes women worry about telling healthcare professionals if they are feeling anxious or depressed because they are worried about being judged as a parent, or think the worst: that their baby will be taken away from them. It really doesn't work like that: supporting a woman and keeping a mum and baby together are always top priority for all professionals. Being open can help prevent depression and anxiety from worsening and ensure that you get the support you need. Please don't be afraid to tell your midwife, health visitor or GP if you think you might be developing any mental health problems. There are specialist teams, psychiatrists like Rebecca, and midwives for managing mental health in pregnancy – which you may be referred to.

These specialists will only want to support you to be the best version of yourself. They will offer a range of other options most suitable for you, from therapy to medication, and you can also find out about local support groups here: www.nhs.uk/service-search/other-services/Mental%20health%20support/ LocationSearch/330.

If you have had a mental health illness in the past, you're more likely to become ill during pregnancy or in the first year after giving birth than at other times in your life. The fluctuating hormones and a general feeling of the unknown can exacerbate existing conditions, so be aware of this and once again, speak to your midwife, GP or health visitor about any current or pre-existing mental health problems: we are there to help you in the best way possible.

WALKING INTO MOTHERHOOD LIKE . . .

You are walking into motherhood and no matter how it presents itself, you'll come out stronger, fiercer and more intuitive. You have got this – trust yourself, your own path and your body. You can always talk to your midwife if you are struggling with any mental health problems; we are here to support you and care for you and your baby.

KEY POINTS

- Your nervous systems are well and truly connected.
- Your baby is learning what it's like to be alive through you.
- Your voice can be heard by your baby.
- Talk to your baby, build a bond with *this* baby at *this* time
- Emotions are chemicals in the blood that can be changed.
- Use steps to manage your emotional wellbeing.
- Talk to your GP or midwife if you are struggling with any mental health issues, as soon as possible.

MATERNITY LEAVE

It might seem early in the book to talk about maternity leave, but you do need to think about it sooner rather than later. Whether you choose to tell your employer right away is up to you; it will depend on how you are feeling and what appointments you need to take, and if they will be during work time. Here are some of the terms you might hear:

Statutory maternity leave is 52 weeks – it's made up of ordinary and additional.

Ordinary maternity leave – first 26 weeks.

Additional maternity leave – last 26 weeks.

The maternity planner found on www.gov.uk/pay-leave-for-parents is really helpful to work out the dates for your ordinary and additional leave. You may also be entitled to take some of your leave as Shared Parental Leave, and if this is something that interests you find out more on www.gov.uk/shared-parental-leave-and-pay. You do not have to take 52 weeks but you must take two weeks' leave after giving birth (or four weeks if you work in a factory).

Maternity leave laws vary around the world, and can vary from woman to woman in the UK too, depending on your work situation. In the UK, during pregnancy you have four main legal rights:

- paid time off for antenatal care
- maternity leave
- maternity pay or maternity allowance
- protection against unfair treatment, discrimination or dismissal

You can take paid time off for antenatal care, and it is worth knowing that this applies to all medical appointments and some antenatal or parenting classes if you've been recommended to attend these by your doctor or midwife.

You could also be entitled to get a one-off payment to help towards the costs of having a baby, known as a Sure Start Maternity Grant. You can ask your midwife for more details about this, but generally, you qualify for the grant if both of the following apply:

- You're expecting your first child, or you're expecting twins and have children already.
- You or your partner already get certain benefits.

You need to claim the grant within 11 weeks of your baby's due date or within six months after your baby's birth.

TELLING YOUR EMPLOYER

Legally, you do need to tell your employer about your pregnancy at least 15 weeks before the beginning of the week the baby is due. You do not need to tell them before then, but if you are going to appointments, it is usually easier to tell them. There may be other considerations you need to make too, such as if you work in an environment that might be detrimental to your health. When you tell your employer about your pregnancy they need to assess any risks to you and your baby. Risks could be caused by things like:

- heavy lifting or carrying
- standing or sitting for long periods without adequate breaks
- exposure to toxic substances
- long working hours

If there are any risks, then your employer needs to take reasonable steps to remove the risks. For example, offering you different work or changing your hours. If your workplace cannot remove any risks then they should agree to let you take a break, on full pay, or they can move you to another role.

Maternity leave and statutory maternity pay will start automatically if you are off work for any pregnancy-related illness in the four weeks before the baby is due and it does not matter what has been previously agreed. Sadly, maternity discrimination is not uncommon worldwide and the UK is no exception. In 2015, an Equality and Human Rights Commission report estimated that 54,000 women a year lose their jobs as a result of maternity discrimination in the UK alone. But the full picture is possibly being masked by the widespread abuse of Non-Disclosure Agreements (NDA).

Social-media influencers (e.g. Joeli @pregnant_then_screwed), charities and mums have made sure government officials are paying attention to the widespread problem of maternity discrimination. MP Maria Millar said in 2019:

'I am proposing a completely new approach with a new law I am presenting to Parliament, the Protection and Maternity (Redundancy Protection) Bill to prohibit redundancy during pregnancy and maternity leave and for six months after the end of the pregnancy or leave, except in specified circumstances. This new law mirrors the approach taken in Germany and has support from members of all the main political parties in Westminster as well as Maternity Action, the charity that campaigns for the rights of pregnant women. With over 15 million women in the UK working and more than 500,000 giving birth every year, we need to make sure that they and their families are supported. Family life and our economy will both suffer unless workplace practices are improved and effective protection against redundancy is an important place to start.'

If you are unsure of your maternity rights and allowance at your work place then you need to speak to your employer or HR department as soon as possible. If you have been a victim of maternity discrimination already, then your first step should be to contact the employment relations organisation ACAS (0300 123 1100); there is also a lot of helpful information on their website for more general questions.

IF YOU'RE SELF-EMPLOYED

To get the full amount of Maternity Allowance, you must have paid Class 2 National Insurance for at least 13 of the 66 weeks before your baby's due. The Department for Work and Pensions (DWP) will check if you've paid enough when you make your claim and they'll write to you if you have not. If you have not paid enough Class 2 National Insurance you'll still get a payment so do ask. You may be able to get the full rate by making extra National Insurance payments. HM Revenue and Customs (HMRC) will send you a letter to tell you how.

Your partner is on a journey too

NOW WE'VE COVERED some of the biggest changes that you face, it is time to shift our attention onto your partner and relationship. This part of the book is about simple ways to help you build strong foundations for your growing family. It is important here that you put a different hat on, just for a minute, and see things from your partner's perspective. I know that not everyone is in a relationship or has a partner, so if this section isn't for you, skip to the next section.

Most of the research into partners during pregnancy is based on dads and men. I know this is not the reality for a lot of couples now, but at the time of writing there is a lack of research into same-sex couples. However, the research we will go into, along with the tips and comments from partners, are helpful for all couples. I hope my intention of helping all couples, in the way that is it meant to, comes across.

Pregnancy is such an important time for your relationship. Now is the time to invest in your relationship to build a strong foundation in preparation for the changes ahead. It's a worthwhile investment because conflict is, more often than not, avoidable. Many couples report experiencing more conflict within the first year after having a baby. I know that may be daunting to hear but that doesn't have to be you. When couples are tired, hormones are in turmoil, tensions are running high and tolerance running low, it is all too easy to slip into a disagreement. You might have to dig deep at times but it is ever so worth it.

Relationship functioning and maternal mental health are also linked. In Diane Speier's book *Life After Birth* she explains that relationship dissatisfaction is one of the strongest indicators for maternal psychological distress. Although

I think there are many factors that affect postnatal mental health and more research (specifically into relationships) is needed, I don't doubt she has a very good point.

Here's a little insider info I've learned. Over the years I asked the couples that appeared to be the happiest and closest what 'the secret' was. I was expecting some huge revelations and real insight but was left surprised at the very simple solutions most of them gave: 'Don't nit-pick' and 'never forget what made you fall in love' were the most common answers. Many couples agreed that bickering was a waste of time and it could cause spirals into unnecessary arguments. I know this is so simple and obvious, but remembering what it is that you really love about your partner may help when you are under strain too.

'Kind words will unlock an iron door'

—TURKISH PROVERB

The most endearing examples of love I have seen are when each partner really empathises with the other and is truly committed to being with them on their journey. The ability to see and feel things from another's perspective is one of our species' most powerful cognitive abilities. This level of empathy goes both ways. Remember that your partner may not be physically pregnant, but s/he will be experiencing all kind of emotions and worries too. They may not want to worry you, but you and your baby are often at the forefront of their mind. Have you ever been in a situation where you need to just stand and observe a loved one do or go through something? Did you almost wish that you could do or go through it for them? Or maybe you got more stressed about it than they did? Having to stand back is a difficult position to be in – feeling helpless is hard to swallow yet it is something most partners feel at some point on their journey.

Partners sometimes get pregnancy symptoms like nausea and hormonal ups and downs too, and it's common for people to laugh at men, especially, who have admitted this. It must be horrible to feel sick and out-of-sorts and then either not be able to admit it or be laughed at if you do. The science backs up these feelings: one study found higher levels of the hormone prolactin and lower levels of testosterone in men who reported two or more pregnancy symptoms like altered appetite, fatigue, nausea and weight gain. Studies in Denmark showed fathers have high levels of anxiety, insecurity and inadequacy during pregnancy that are not addressed because the focus is on mum and baby.

New Macho is a company that is dedicated to help brands grow through creating a new male narrative. Their recent research and findings have clearly shown how harmful stereotypes can be. I spoke to Fernando Desouches, the managing director and father of two, to find out more about his mission and personal experience:

'Becoming a father is one of the biggest transformations that money can't buy. I'm a father of two sons and started New Macho (the specialised marketing-to-men arm of the brand and cultural transformation company, BBD Perfect Storm) when I realised how many men are performing the life that is expected for them to live instead of being and acting as who they really are. I believe that brand communications can play a fundamental role in helping men to define a new aspiration that serves them, rather than adding pressure.

'There are several changes, physical and psychological, that affect men when their first baby is born. Lack of sleep and increased responsibilities are the ones we might be more aware of, but other major changes also happen. There is a reduction in the level of fathers' testosterone; we start an unconscious process of identification with our own fathers. This in turn can connect us to 'unfinished business' that might arise.

'Additionally, the increase in caring responsibility is magnified by the lack of a "rite of passage for men" in our society. Nobody teaches us how to become adult men and many men are not psychologically ready to deal with this change. In the best cases of this situation, fathers are forced to learn by doing.

'With these considerations, it is not surprising that 70 per cent of men report feeling increased stress when they become fathers for the first time. Another tricky factor is that one in four also feel isolated during the first 12 months (source: Movember Foundation). Men talk less than women about their mental health issues and are less inclined to seek help. Many men feminise the idea of taking care of themselves or asking for support; they think it is the mark of a man to deal with his own sh*t.

'In this case, we all need help and it would be great to normalise this message. This would reduce the stress and achieve better connections between men and their families in the first year of the new baby to make it an even more enjoyable experience. In the first stage, preparatory messaging targeting future fathers, targeting them around all the emotions to come. Additionally, employers should play a role in facilitating more flexible paternity leave policies, supported with messaging to encourage first-time dads to talk to relatives and/or experts if needed.

'But at the same time, becoming a father can be a fantastic opportunity for men to reconnect with their sense of purpose: What is the legacy he wants to leave for his son/daughter? It's time to see the big picture and reconnect with who we really are, with our values, and what we do, or can do, to live them.'

I know it is a long-standing sort of joke about men having no idea what it is really like, but although this is true, it does have limitations and they are very much on a journey too. Your midwife is an advocate for you – the word midwife literally means 'with woman' – but I also think it is time we all addressed and listened to how a lot of partners feel. Here are a few more quotes from some of my friends about how they really felt during pregnancy and at the birth:

'I was worried that I wouldn't be able to help her enough because I wasn't going through what she was. At times I felt distant because I didn't know things that she knew about the baby. I remember one time I asked to feel the baby kicking and she said "she's asleep". I don't know why but I felt hurt in a way. I think she thought I wasn't that excited, but I just felt kind of silly for asking so I didn't any more.'

First-time dad and husband of a midwife

'Every appointment I went to I was pretty much ignored. It was almost like I did my bit by getting her pregnant – then I was ignored. I'd do it all again and I know it's not about me, it just felt like my presence wasn't needed and I wasn't really a part of the conversations or asked much. Then at the birth I was expected to know what to do and I just didn't. I wish I had spoken up about how I felt more, but typical bloke, I didn't feel like I could say.'

First-time dad

'Towards the end of the pregnancy I was worried that something would happen to my girlfriend and the baby, but I didn't want to worry her, so I didn't say how I felt. That was one of the hardest parts, trying to be her rock and also hide that I was really worried.'

First-time mum

WHAT YOU CAN BOTH DO

Talking to your partner about their feelings benefits you both in the long run. Check in often with your other half, and ask them how they are feeling about the pregnancy, birth and becoming a parent, because this can give them the opportunity they may need to let you know how they are feeling. Think of it like a flight: you can't get on board without checking in, and you both need to be 'on board' the flight. Studies have shown that when partners are educated and involved, postnatal depression is reduced and breastfeeding is more successful. Communication is the anchor of any kind of human interaction. We all know how a few simple words can completely change a person's whole state of mind.

'Words are the most powerful drug known to man'

— KIPLING

YOUR PARTNER'S INVOLVEMENT

Something that really helps with partner involvement is attending appointments. Encourage your partner to come to as many appointments as possible. That way they are up to date so communication and planning are far easier for the both of you. The appointment is also a chance for them to ask questions. When I ask partners if they have questions, quite often they do. They just need someone to address them, so they feel able to say what is on their mind. If the midwife doesn't ask your partner directly, then you can perhaps ask if they have any questions before you leave. The quote from a dad that felt like he was not important or needed is sad, and may have impacted on his early experience of fatherhood. Even if your partner doesn't have any questions, the fact that someone is listening and addressing them changes the whole dynamic of the conversation.

> 'Whether the partner is male or female is completely irrelevant as long as they are supportive.'
>
> — DR THOMAS VERNY, PSYCHIATRIST

Being at the appointments means your partner will be able to hear your baby's heartbeat and see the scans. Any mystery is reduced, and can help the partner feel more at ease, connected, but most importantly *involved*. The feeling of involvement is essential for bonding.

You know when you've not spoken to an old friend for a while and then she calls and asks 'how are you, what's happening?' It's kind of hard to answer because you aren't sure where to start. If your partner doesn't come to appointments regularly, they can slip out of the loop and only get slices of information. Your partner may also be able to help you after the appointment if you've forgotten something at a later date; it's another set of ears.

I know it may not be realistic for your partner to be able to come to every single appointment, but the most important ones are the scans so they can physically see your baby moving and see their little hands and toes. The 25-week (if it is your first) or 28-week (if you have had a baby before) appointment is also a good one to attend, because you will hear your baby' heartbeat, your tummy will be measured and you can see your baby's growth together. Lastly, the 36-week appointment is usually when your birth plan will be discussed, and if your partner plans to be at the birth, this one is so useful to attend.

If work commitments are an issue, you can always ask your midwife about appointment times that are more suitable for your partner; some clinics are held on a weekend. Legally, the minimum amount of unpaid leave a partner is entitled to is two appointments each lasting up to 6.5 hours. After that they can take annual leave or request further unpaid leave. It is rare that employers are difficult at this time, but if taking time off is becoming an issue you need to liaise with ACAS (see page 82). Let your partner do this because you don't want/need the hassle. If your partner really can't make appointments, then why not record your baby's heartbeat for them to hear later?

If you decide to go to antenatal classes, taking your partner makes the world of difference. First of all, they get the heads-up on what to expect, secondly they can really help you make decisions about what you want and support you, and thirdly they also get to meet other partners who are expecting. No longer is pregnancy and birth 'women's business' that partners are ushered away from. Knowing what to expect and how to prepare helps them to help you. When you or your midwife talk about things like pain relief or colostrum, they will know what you mean and won't feel left out of the conversation or silly for not knowing. It is also good for your partner to socialise, couples tend to bond and meet up outside of the classes too. I know couples that met at antenatal classes ten years ago and still holiday together today.

Another thing that can help is buying and choosing things for the baby together. Suggest that your partner picks out an outfit for the baby. This may be the only time your partner actually enjoys going shopping with you! It is so exciting and makes it more real for your partner too. They need to think about all the practicalities of having a newborn, what is needed, and how to use products as well as you do. A lot of shops give parents demonstrations and safety advice on things like car seats or prams, so if you buy these items together, they will also know how to use the kit they will also be using regularly. You may have a lot on your mind, so once again it's an extra pair of ears and shared decision-making.

Lastly, invest in time together; have date nights and set aside time to just spend on each other. It doesn't need to be anything extravagant, even just a weekly exercise routine, sitting at the table and dedicating times to eat and catch up or regular evening stroll together is enough. This is a lot easier when it is your first baby, but it is still important to dedicate time to each other if you already have children. Asking your partner to do something with you makes them feel valued too. They can feel a bit left out or less important during pregnancy, especially when the focus is on you and the baby. By no means am I suggesting that the focus shouldn't be on you, it should, but it is important to remember your partner is also going through a major life change. They need to process their emotions and may be anxious, worried or uncertain about how to help. When you catch up regularly you understand each other better.

LET'S TALK ABOUT SEX, BABY . . .

Let's cut to the chase – yes, sex is safe for the majority of women. Your baby is protected by your cervix, mucus plug (sounds grim, but it is a really helpful guard) and the amniotic sack – your waters. If you have been told you have a cervical erosion (cells that are normally inside cervix are seen on the outside too) or any changes to your cervix, this can cause some spotting (drops of blood) after sex. To make sure it is safe for you, ask your midwife or doctor. If your waters have broken, or if you are in a polygamous relationship, then you need to avoid sex to reduce the risk of infection. Lastly, if you are at risk of pre-term labour, you should avoid sex too.

The truth about sex during pregnancy is that every woman is different. Some women's sex drive completely changes and they think about or want sex all the time – the significant increase in blood flow to the pelvic region may explain the sudden accelerated sex drive. My friend told me that for the first time in their marriage her husband had to 'turn me down because *he* was too tired!' Other women want more sexual encounters but not penetrative sex. And for some, the thought of sex makes them want to vomit. All of these reactions are normal. Whether or not you want sex is down to a range of things like hormones, how you feel about your body, if you have pelvic pain, and how pregnant you are. Not wanting sex is not a reflection of how you feel about your partner and usually your sex drives returns when you are ready.

Position-wise, see what is most comfortable for you, but the spooning position is popular. It seems to be the most comfortable for everything: boobs, bump and pelvis.

IF THERE'S A PROBLEM . . .

I know this section has all been about bonding, love and seeing things from your partner's point of view, but I also need to be honest with you about abusive behaviour. The majority of partners are caring, and this section in the book may well help to support all of their positive traits. However, sadly it is well known that domestic abuse increases, and can even start, during pregnancy, more than at any other time. Victim Support UK recently revealed that 30 per cent of domestic violence cases occur for the first time in pregnancy. Always remember that midwives and healthcare professionals are here to help and support you. We are here to protect you and we really care about you and your baby's wellbeing. Professionals won't judge you so please don't feel embarrassed to come to us. You will not be the first or last to tell us, and domestic abuse can happen to *anyone*. If you're scared of your partner or what they might do, please do not wait to tell your midwife as there are many people who can help too: emergency contacts are REACH 0800 088 4194 or National Domestic Abuse Helpline 0808 200 0247.

KEY POINTS

- Invest in, and build your family foundations during pregnancy.
- Your partner is on their own journey too, so try and be mindful of that.
- Coming to appointments matters and you *both* have a legal right to time off.
- Your relationship is important. Communicate, catch up and dedicate time to each other.
- Acknowledge and act upon any abnormal behaviour. Midwives are always here to help, as well as many other people. You are never alone.

Birth is unpredictable – why plan?

PEOPLE SOMETIMES SAY, 'Birth is unpredictable, so don't plan in case you get disappointed.' If that were true would anyone ever make a plan for anything? We *generally* don't think, 'Well, I better not plan for that just in case I get disappointed if it doesn't work out.' We have wedding plans, business plans, holiday plans, and some of us have five-year plans, so why not plan and properly prepare for birth too? You are a strong woman – you know your own body and your mind – so let's make a plan for how you would like your birth to go. And yes, it should be called a plan. Some people are now recommending we ditch the word plan and use 'preference' instead, but you won't hear any other leader saying, 'Our preference is to ensure we build 100 more schools by 2025.' They would say exactly what they *plan* for, even if they are not sure they will achieve it. As you are the leader and make the final decisions, it is important that you own it and have a plan.

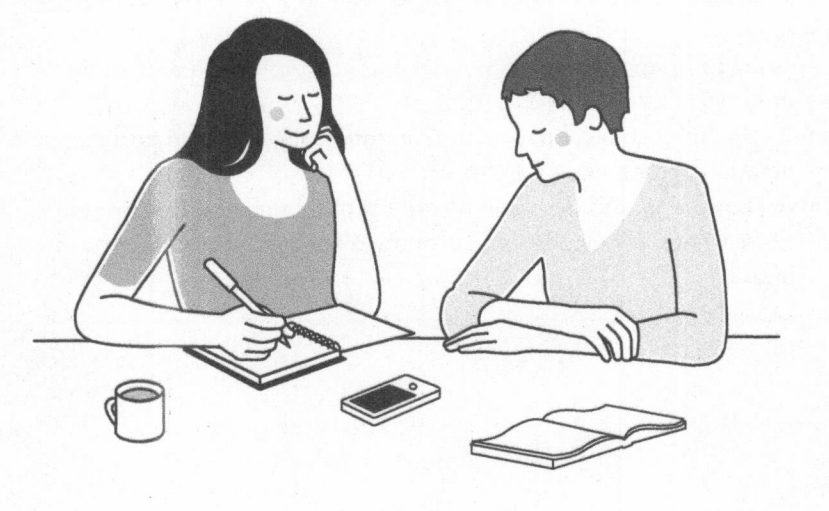

It is true that birth is unpredictable but that doesn't mean you have no control over what happens. It doesn't mean that you don't need to know about your options, or just 'go with the flow', and it doesn't mean that when one thing doesn't go according to plan it all has to go out the window – you can have plans A, B and C ready to go. We will never be able to control uncertainty so we might as well plan to work with that, and part of planning the unpredictable is knowing what your options are. This section will explain how to do just that and a bit about what all birth plans should have.

MAKING YOUR PLAN

Understanding how birth works, knowing what you want, and letting those caring for you also know what you want, leads to a more positive birth experience. The only way to be in control is by knowing what you want. That said, you shouldn't ignore a recommendation you are given by your healthcare professional; it is important to weigh it all up (see page 38).

A VISUAL BIRTH PLAN

You can now make a visual birth plan that uses pictures rather than words.

Little visuals give everyone more information quickly, which is especially helpful when women are in the zone or labour is advancing quickly. It can help your midwife too, as they are quicker to check.

You can download a Visual Birthplan at: themodernmidwife.com/visual-birthplan.

Making a plan is typically done at your 36-week appointment but check with your midwife when you need to make a plan. Ideally, your birth partner should be with you when you do your birth plan and should also go through it with your midwife. Having your birth partner there is important because it allows them to be a true advocate for you. Most of the time I communicate more with the birth partner than I do with the woman in labour. Women in established labour (see page 199 for more on the stages of labour) don't usually want to have a conversation, but there may be some additional questions I need to ask. It is like a breath of fresh air when the birth partner can give such important information. The birth partner and I can really work as a little team together. It's a much better experience for everyone.

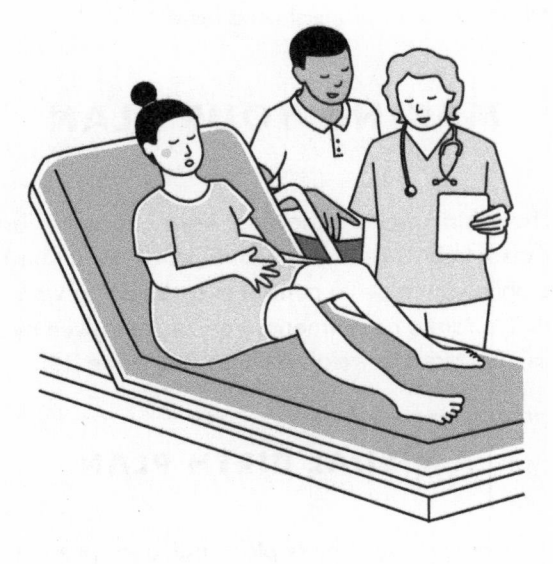

Birth plans themselves vary massively, from home water birth to a planned C-section. Whatever you plan there are key things you need to consider.

WHERE DO YOU WANT TO GIVE BIRTH?

By 36 weeks, your pregnancy is usually progressed enough for you and your midwife to decide where it is safest for you to give birth. The options are usually:

- At home. This is suitable for low-risk pregnancies and particularly suitable for women who have had a baby before with no complications. You'll need to hire a pool if you want a water birth.

- In a stand-alone midwifery-led unit. This is a unit in its own right that is not attached to a hospital. A team of midwives will provide all the care a woman and her baby need. Birth pools are usually provided. If a transfer to hospital is needed then an ambulance will be required (even though most transfers are not emergencies).
- A midwifery-led unit in hospital. These are usually attached to a labour ward or very close by. If a transfer to the hospital labour ward is needed it's a case of being wheeled across. Birth pools are usually provided.
- Labour ward/delivery suite, in hospital. Most suitable for women with medical conditions or pregnancy complications. The labour ward is also the only place an epidural can be done.

Your midwife will use evidence-based information to help you choose what is most suitable for you and your baby.

I have been at some incredibly beautiful, calm home births. Being in the comfort of your own home can have such a positive impact on not only the natural workings of your body but also your experience of labour and birth. The first few hours after birth are so undisturbed and peaceful. Helping a woman into her own bed with a cuppa after having a baby is priceless.

'There's no place like home ...'

—DOROTHY, *THE WIZARD OF OZ*

In the UK, many women safely opt for a home birth, and we are ever so lucky to have access to medical care should we need it. Experienced midwives are very good at preventing and managing change or deviation from the norm. When things 'go wrong' they *usually* do so slowly, leaving us time to get extra help or transfer into hospital. The best evidence we have shows that home birth for healthy 'low-risk' women, overall, means less intervention and better outcomes for both first-time mums and for women that have had babies before. Home birth appears to be safer for *all* low-risk women.

If this is your first baby, there is some evidence to show that home birth is less safe for babies, though, as there is a very small increase in 'adverse outcome' of babies of first-time mums. A midwifery-led unit is the next best option, because the rate of intervention is lower and the outcome for the baby is no different compared with an obstetric unit (labour ward).

The bullets below outline some of the common conditions that increase risk and lead to women being advised against a homebirth.

- If your body mass index (BMI) is greater than 35.
- If your baby is not cephalic (head down).
- If your baby is small for gestational age.
- If you go into labour before 37 weeks.
- If you have developed a condition in pregnancy such as pre-eclampsia, gestational diabetes or high blood pressure.
- If you have had episodes of bleeding in pregnancy.
- If you have had a Caesarean section before.
- If you have a long-standing medical condition
- If you are having twins or more.

It is worth saying that if you are aged over 35 (the age of recommended individual assessment as stated by NICE), there is no suggestion that *all* women over 35 should be advised against a home birth. So, if you are 37 years old, very healthy, exercise, have no medical conditions, no complications during pregnancy, and have easy access to a hospital, then home birth is likely to be as safe as it is for a 35-year-old. You need to look at the whole picture rather than one risk factor.

If you have been advised against a home birth, but you think it should still be an option for you, then you need to request to talk to the Midwifery Matron or Head of Midwifery at your hospital about your individual options, and what is safest and best for both you and your baby. It is important to openly discuss your options, your personal risks and benefits each step of the way, so you feel comfortable with what you're doing and why. You never want to feel as though you are being forced to go somewhere or have had an opportunity taken away from you. Your planned place of birth should be a shared decision, based on your personal circumstances and the latest evidence, so you have your baby in the safest place possible and feel happy about that.

WHO SHOULD YOU BRING WITH YOU?

～～～

You need to decide who your birth tribe will be. If you are on the labour ward or at a Midwifery-led unit, it is usually recommended that you have a maximum of two birth partners. If you have a home birth you can have whoever you like – as long as it is safe and easy to move around. See page 188 for more on choosing your birth partners. Write their names on your birth plan; it is so helpful for midwives when women name those that are with them in their birth plan; knowing who is who gives you a better connection. 'Is it Andy?' is so much more welcoming than, 'Sorry, I didn't catch your name?' if you have not met before.

Your birth partner has an extremely important role in helping, supporting and caring for you, so tell them exactly what is important to you at your birth and go through the birth plan with them, if you have not done so already.

It is also helpful for us to know whether or not you mind having students at your birth, so put that on the plan too. That way we don't need to interrupt your labour to ask.

WHAT ABOUT PAIN RELIEF MEDICATION?

～～～

No matter where or how you labour and birth, there will be pain relief options. At home or in a midwifery-led unit, generally you can have most of what we offer in hospital other than an epidural. There are many forms of pain management that are drug-free, such as: natural pain relief released by the body when you're in 'the zone', hydrotherapy, aromatherapy, using a birthing ball, TENS machine, massage, breathing exercises, hypnobirthing, mental reframing, support from your tribe and midwife, environment and visualisations etc., and most of these work best if you've been practising during pregnancy. We will go into your birthing body and create a unique toolkit for you in the next section (see page 166). A lot of women ask what medication they can have and what each do, so I have created a list below. The medication for pain relief varies between hospitals but to give you an idea most hospitals offer these – starting with the least invasive:

- **Oral analgesia:** These include paracetamol, dihydrocodeine or sometimes oral morphine. These usually take around 20 minutes to kick in and wear off after 4–6 hours, depending on the dose given and how quickly your body metabolises it. Opioids cross the placenta, so your baby does receive a small amount of this drug.
- **Gas and air:** Also known as Entonox, or by the nickname 'laughing gas', and I've had some serious laughs with women using this. One night shift, I'll never forget it, a woman had me in stitches; we were both howling with laughter and seeing the funny side to everything. Her husband came back from the car like ... 'what the hell is going on with you two?' We'd lost it and I wasn't even using the gas (obvs)! The gas is inhaled and is quickly metabolised so works pretty much instantly; it is usually used later on in labour and is not recommended before you're in established labour. It is not believed to cross the placenta so your baby doesn't receive any. The downside is that it can cause nausea and/or vomiting, especially if used for long periods of time. The good news is that it is very short-lasting so any side effects wear off quickly.
- **Injection:** This is usually pethidine, which is opioid-based. An injection takes about 20 minutes to start working. Usually you can have two doses prescribed by a midwife and generally the third dose needs to be prescribed by a doctor, but hospital protocols vary. You can have the injections two to three hours apart. These medications can often make women vomit or feel sick, so we offer an anti-sickness medication in with the injection. You may feel spaced out and even get some sleep after having pethidine. I have seen it work wonders for some women and not work at all for others. Some midwives say they think it works best in the latent phase (less than 4cm dilated and contracting irregularly) because it can relax you at this time. It does cross the placenta and is safest when given more than two hours before birth. If your baby is born within two hours of the injection it can cause your baby to be a little sleepy at birth and be slow to feed so it's best to have pethidine earlier on to reduce the risk of a sleepy baby.
- **Epidural:** This is when a needle is used to insert a small plastic tube called an epidural catheter between the bones of your back, the needle is removed and the catheter stays in that space. Anaesthetic (pain

relief) medication is then administered via this catheter. An epidural can only be done by an anaesthetic doctor in a hospital setting. Most NHS hospitals do not have 'walking epidurals' yet, so you will most likely need to be on a bed. That doesn't mean you have to sit on your back the whole time (see page 207 for more info). Because an epidural has side effects such as a drop in blood pressure, you will need to be cannulated (have a little tube in a hand vein via a needle) for fluids to be given. All hospitals recommend monitoring of your baby's heartbeat after epidural, because drugs from the epidural can affect babies and occasionally they get distressed (show a change in heart rate.) This is most common when you have the first dose of the epidural, even though the heartbeat usually returns to normal very quickly; it is important to monitor.

DO I NEED TO PLAN FOR THE CORD AND PLACENTA?

~~~

Your baby is connected to you via the cord and placenta so you need to think about these when making your birth plan.

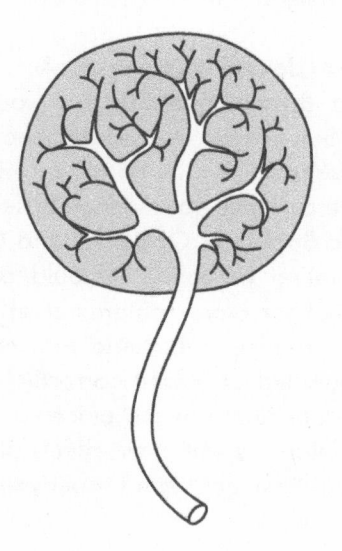

First up, the cord. Delaying clamping and cutting the cord by a *minimum* of one minute after birth is recommended. This gives your baby up to 30 per cent more oxygen, iron and nutrient-rich blood compared to immediate clamping and cutting. Delayed cord clamping is generally standard practice now, but it's still worth putting this in your birth plan alongside who you want to do this life-changing deed! Cutting the cord marks the moment your baby becomes independent from you. You, your birth partner or your midwife can cut the cord.

Then you need to think about your placenta. As you know it is a very special and unique organ. The main things you need to consider about it are:

1. Do you want an injection to help deliver your placenta? (We refer to delivering the placenta as the third stage of labour).
   An injection to encourage the placenta to come out will be offered to you whether you are at risk of bleeding or not. If you are at an increased risk, your midwife will explain why this is recommended. The injection can reduce initial blood loss and speed the delivery of the placenta, however, it can make you feel nauseous, especially if you have had an otherwise drug-free birth. The other option is to have a physiological third stage, where you let your body do it naturally and have drugs if you need them. Putting the baby on your breast and having a wee are also natural ways of also encouraging the placenta to come out.

2. What do you want to do with your placenta?
   This may seem a strange question and you may not want to do anything with it. But to give you some ideas: Are you keeping it? Burying it? Encapsulating it? It is up to you what you do, but bear in mind that there are currently no evidence-based benefits of consuming your placenta. The Society of Obstetrics and Gynaecologists Canada reported encapsulating or eating it could cause harm to mothers due to the potential for cross-contamination and transfer of blood-borne pathogens (a virus or bacteria that can make you ill) if the placenta is not handled or stored correctly. Although iron, oxytocin and progesterone are found in the placenta, their maintenance and stability in preparation, as well their effects after consumption on the postpartum woman, have not been properly tested yet.

3. Do you want to see your placenta/or not?

Personally, I think the veins leading to the cord on your baby's side are worth seeing; they look a bit like roots to a tree and are smooth in texture, and seeing this leaves you able to picture how your baby was kept alive inside you and also how big the wound inside you is as the placenta has come away from the lining of your uterus. The initial blood loss you are getting usually comes from where the placenta has been. But not everyone agrees with me on the importance of seeing the placenta – some people are a little more squeamish and don't want to see it. It is always your choice!

THE PAUSE

Immediately once you have given birth to your baby, there comes what is called 'the pause'. The birth pause is rarely talked about, so for all the info you need on that head to page 224. For the purpose of your birth plan you need to have a think about the moment you meet your baby. Some women like to leave their baby where they 'land', so to speak; this may be just underneath you on a bed, or in the arms of a midwife. It is not at all uncommon to not want to hold your baby right away. Pausing for a minute is instinctive and most women just need a minute or so to go from pushing power to stopping, to then slowly meeting their baby. Something incredibly powerful just happened and has permanently changed your life, so it's only natural that you may need to catch your breath first.

WHAT'S VITAMIN K?

In the UK, vitamin K is recommened as an injection to all newborns at birth because it is most effective when administered now. An alternative is oral drops (generally four doses over one week or one month, but this varies.) Some babies develop a rare and unpredictable disorder called Vitamin K Deficiency Bleeding (VKDB) and babies affected can bleed from various places, but most concerning they can get a brain haemorrhage as a result of this condition.

VKDB can therefore lead to brain damage and in very rare cases, death. We can't predict what babies will suffer with VKDB which is why all babies are offered vitamin K as a preventative measure.

WHAT IF I NEED A C-SECTION?

This may sound like really odd advice, especially if you are planning a natural birth, but you do need to consider Caesarean sections on your birth plan. A C-section can be life-saving surgery and I want to be 100 per cent honest with you – some babies become distressed during labour, or things change, and a C-section is what is needed to keep you and/or your baby safe. There are many things you can do to optimise your environment, stay active and manage pain, and there are positions you can get into to help speed your labour up and help your baby come through your pelvis with ease. I don't doubt any of your body's natural abilities. However, knowledge is power. You don't need to fixate on the possibility of having a C-section but understanding the basics make it less scary and far easier to accept at the time. Here is what usually happens:

- You will be seen by an anaesthetist who will run through some standard questions with you and recommend that you have a cannula in your hand (to get access to your vein for medication and fluids, if needed).
- The anaesthetist's main job is to make sure that you are comfortable during the procedure and they will put in (site) and administer the spinal. If you have already had an epidural, sometimes they can manage with this. The anaesthetist will be mostly with you at the 'head end' so you'll see a lot of their face.
- Only one other person is able to come into theatre with you, so have a think now about who you might want if you have more than one birth partner. Your midwife will be with you, too.
- The theatre team can look quite daunting as there can be around seven people, but they all have their special jobs. It's normal to have a theatre team for any operation.
- You'll need a catheter to collect your wee as you won't be mobile. Since there can be a lot of people in theatre you can request for

other staff to be at your head end; they don't need to observe you having a catheter put in. Usually the midwife will do this for you, so if you feel more comfortable you can ask her to direct the room for you. It is important that you are at the centre of your care and these very simple things matter because they protect your dignity. If you don't care that is also fine but you don't need to leave your dignity at the door; I don't care what anyone says – yes, your most private and intimate parts may be exposed but you don't have to become powerless and exposed unnecessarily. In a true emergency everyone will need to focus on getting the best outcome and work at a faster pace, but unless this is the case, we can all work to ensure you and your body are respected and treated with dignity throughout.

- The obstetrician will be the person doing your C-section and if you have any requests put this on your birth plan. For example, you can ask for the drape (between your head and your tummy) to be lowered so you can see as doctor slowly delivers your baby with gentle pressure. We sometimes call this a 'woman-centred' or 'gentle C-section'. You can also put on your plan that you want the monitors on your back or side rather than your chest so that you can have skin-to-skin contact with your baby as soon as possible, and if you aren't feeling up to it your birth partner can. It is the obstetrician who can facilitate this. Of course, if your baby needs to be born very quickly or be seen by a paediatrician, you wouldn't want to put yourself or your baby in danger, and some of these options may not be possible, but most of the time they are and it is important to put on your plan what you want.
- Once you have had your baby, you will be taken to a 'recovery' room where a midwife or nurse will be with you, do your observations for a bit, and check you over a few times.
- If you want to breastfeed and you haven't yet, then you should try to feed your baby as soon as possible. Sometimes that is still in theatre. The midwife can help you do this and recommend good positions for you as you will want to avoid any pressure on your tummy.
- Depending on how you are feeling, after an hour or so, you should be offered some tea and toast – a bliss moment!
- If your baby needs to go to special care, please don't think that you can't do all the things you planned for right away. You can have postponed

skin-to-skin, cuddles and kisses; it is just as precious and important that you still do these things and don't consider them to be lost.

'I would just like every belly birth mum to know that she can have a birth that she can be in control of! Of course it's dependent on the level of emergency but it can still be a positive experience. Some women honestly don't know that the drape can be lowered, or that the partner can cut the cord ... With both births I had a belly birth plan, so that in that occasion the team know what points are important to you!'

Heidi, second-time mum

ASSISTED BIRTH

There are other possibilities that you may be offered, such as forceps or ventouse, where an obstetrician will help your baby be born. Forceps are metal tongs that look a bit like salad servers and ventouse is a little cap placed on your baby's head that creates a suction to guide your baby out. These are most commonly recommended when your baby is low down in your pelvis and is able to be born vaginally but when there is a need to speed up the birth. They are used if your baby has become distressed, you have become tired from pushing or are unable to push, or your baby is in a difficult position. Most of the time the doctor will need to do an episiotomy (a small cut at an angle to your perineum to create more room). This will then be sutured (stitched) after birth. Although these may sound a bit scary, some women say that they gained great relief from this help and would have it again. Other women don't have such a positive experience as there is an increased risk of perineal trauma and incontinence after birth. For this reason, some women put in their birth plan that they would prefer a C-section to an assisted birth. It is good to have a think about this but perhaps assess at the time. Some assisted births are more gentle and calm and others can be more difficult depending on the unique situation. No matter what happens, always remember and refer back to your BRAIN tool, ask questions and stick as closely as possible to the other plans you have.

PLANNING FOR THE BIRTH

Ultimately your birth should contain all of these elements. If you plan for them now, and understand what they are, then you are doing all you can to make them happen.

- Preparation and understanding
- A safe, caring environment
- A supportive birth partner
- Professional, unbiased support
- You in control
- Use of breathing and relaxation techniques
- Trust in those caring for you
- Options and alternatives
- Informed choice and shared decision-making
- Protected time for you and your baby
- Delayed cord clamping
- Skin-to-skin at the earliest time possible

Remember that your birth plan can change at any time and having a plan A, B and C allows you to be open and flexible to changing your mind at any time. You will make the best choice for you at the time. Try to let go of 'right' and 'wrong' as you're making these decisions. Until you're experiencing labour, you may not have all the answers, but there is no doubt in my mind that it is best to go in with a plan and create an environment that works with you and your body's natural physiology.

KEY POINTS

- Some situations are out of our control but we can plan to work with them by being educated on the options and possibilities.
- Understand how birth works, know what you want, and communicate it in a written or visual plan.
- A birth plan is just that – a plan. It's not written in stone and you can deviate from it if you want.
- Have a think about plan A, B and C – what do you want if your plan needs to deviate?
- Let go of 'right' and 'wrong' as you make decisions; you will do what is best for you and your baby at the time.

Preparing for birth

THERE ARE LOTS of things you can do to prepare for the birth, from planning how to get to hospital, to making sure you have practised birthing positions. In this section, we will run through the areas that I get asked about most.

HELPING YOUR BABY INTO THE BEST POSITION

It might seem early to think about this, but you can start thinking about getting your baby into position weeks before the actual birth. There are some really simple and easy things you can do to help your baby get into the best position for labour and birth. From 34 weeks ask your midwife about what position your baby is in because your baby's position is a key part of having a quicker and easier labour. Your baby needs to have as much space at the front of your pelvis as possible so that they can face your spine. This is called occiput anterior, meaning the smallest part of your baby's head is coming first; and why labour and birth can be a little easier and shorter.

Wherever you sit the most, whether at work, or at home, pop a cushion underneath your bottom to tilt and raise your pelvis above your knees. Have a cushion in the car too, if you drive a lot. Aim to be upright, slightly forward, and have your legs open; this is known as the UFO (upright, forward, open) position.

BABY IN
OCCIPUT-ANTERIOR
(OA) POSITION, WITH
THEIR FACE TOWARDS
YOUR SPINE

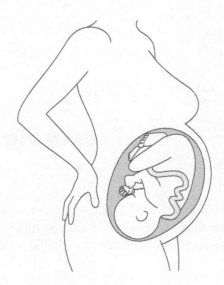

All-fours is also a good position to help baby gravitate around to the anterior position (although you might want to save that one for home rather than in the office). Here are some more tips for helping to get baby into position:

- Sit on a birthing ball or a bean bag if you are watching TV, rather than slouch back on the sofa. You might like to kneel over a bean bag to vary this.
- When you sit on an upright chair, place your feet flat on the floor and lean forward (your belly will hang between your knees.)
- If you sit a lot, take regular breaks, get up and move around.
- Swim on your front but avoid breaststroke if you have pelvic pain; instead you can use a float or hold onto the side of the pool and stretch your legs out behind you.

All of these help to prepare you for an active birth and also allow you to experiment with ways that you feel most comfortable when encouraging your baby to get into a good position for birth. For example, in pregnancy some women have been going onto all-fours at home and they naturally get into this position when they are ready to push – it's like they instinctively know that is how they need to be to help their baby come through their pelvis. If your baby is in the OP position please don't worry, that doesn't mean your labour is doomed. Most babies turn in labour – especially if you are active.

'Active birth is a combination of exercising during pregnancy, feeling informed and confident through antenatal education, and using upright and active positions during birth. Active birth techniques are really empowering for women and help to facilitate a sense of control and promote physiological birth. The evidence suggests that in the first stage of labour, being upright and mobile can reduce the length of labour, the need for a Caesarean birth or an epidural, and babies are less likely to be admitted to the neonatal unit. Upright positions used in the second stage of labour can reduce the length of this stage, the need for assisted births and episiotomies and cause less distress for babies. So get practising! Feel confident about yourself – you're growing a baby! Move your incredible body, research your options, remember to breathe, and lastly don't be afraid to take charge!'

Cheryl Samuels, NHS Midwife, Instagram @the_holistic_midwife, Team member @bloodtobaby

PRACTISE USING A BIRTH BALL

A birthing ball can help to utilise and create space in your pelvis and encourage your baby to get into the best position for labour and birth. Research shows that birthing balls can also reduce lower back pain in late pregnancy and in labour.

Several studies reveal that birthing balls reduce the average length of labour. Interestingly, there is also a link between using a birthing ball and reduction in the need for a C-section in first-time mums. Links aren't absolute proof, but they are worth taking note of.

Birthing balls encourage pelvic relaxation and rhythmic movement (which can be hard to maintain during labour). This movement activates the right side of the brain and encourages the physical rather than the cerebral. Basically, it really helps take your mind off things because your brain struggles to process both sides of thinking at the same time.

Things to try with your ball during labour are:

1. Bounce on your ball.
2. Rotate one way, then the other.
3. Stretch out one leg, leaning to one side then the other.
4. Kneel with your knees apart and lean over your ball with your arms.

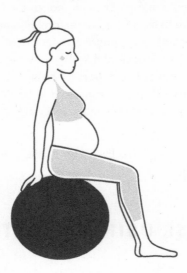

To get the most out of using a birthing ball, make sure that you use it regularly in pregnancy from the third trimester and get comfy with it. Try watching TV on it or using it at work. Some of the pregnant midwives I have worked with (who have office-based roles) bring their birthing ball to work and sit on it instead of a chair – this might not be suitable for all workplaces but is something to consider, especially if you work from home.

WHAT TO PACK IN YOUR LABOUR BAG

Whether you are planning a home or a hospital birth you will need to pack a labour bag and have it ready by about 37 weeks – although some women like to pack sooner. There are endless lists online with what to pack ... sometimes I read these and think, 'What the ...?' Ask any second-time mum about the difference between her first and second labour bag ... If you end up staying longer than planned you can always get someone to top you up with clothes etc. Here is the no-nonsense list of what I'd pack for myself, starting with what you need for baby, and then what you need for you:

Nappies: As these will be on your baby's skin for the best part of 24 hours a day, seven days a week, you may want to consider what product to buy and how this may affect your baby. Each child uses around 8,000 nappies and regular disposable nappies can take up to 100 years to degrade in landfill, or end up in an incinerator. Biodegradable nappies usually have fewer chemicals in them, and are made from more natural fibres, which are good for both your baby and better for the environment – although the jury is still out on how well they degrade. Washable nappies are another option; have a think about what works best for your family and the future environmental impact. There are too many variables for me to give conclusive advice on what is best for every family.

Babywear: You'll need a couple of vests, a couple of babygrows, one body suit and one hat to leave hospital in. Your baby has been in a natural and safe environment in the womb, so if you can, try to opt for organic cotton babywear for the first four weeks, if possible, and pre-wash them in bicarbonate of soda (rinse well). This is kinder to their skin and helps reduce some unnecessary exposure to the chemicals found in clothes manufacturing and washing detergents. Boy or girl, cream or white colour is best; if you have never had the pleasure of dealing with a poo explosion you're in for a treat. What comes out of your tiny baby can be rather impressive – and get everywhere. You can boil wash cream/white clothing and get the poo stains out rather than ruin outfit after outfit. Try and opt for babywear that fastens down the front as it's so much easier to get on.

Muslins: These fabric squares are just brilliant and versatile, from mopping up sick, protecting your shoulder whilst winding, to a little blanket or wrap. You are guaranteed to make use of a muslin or two.

Cotton wool: For the first few days of life, your baby will pass meconium, a type of poo, which is thick, black and sticky (a bit like Marmite). It can be difficult to clean off. Using baby wipes can strip the all-important skin barriers, and the cold sensation of a wipe is not pleasant for a newborn. You will need to keep rubbing the same section of skin to remove the meconium and this can become very sore for your newborn. Warm water and cotton wool is all you need in those early days.

Formula: If you plan to bottle-feed your baby, you will need to take some formula and bottles with you, otherwise don't worry about getting formula. Formula milk in most high-street shops is manufactured by the same companies. They all need to stick to the same strict guidelines, so the truth of the matter is, they all look different due to marketing and packaging, but they are all very similar.

And that's all you really need for your newborn. They don't care how much you have bought them or what anyone else thinks. They just want as many comforts as possible – usually provided by you and skin-to-skin contact.

Your antenatal notes: Unless your hospital has gone digital, your notes are key. They have got everything we need to know about you, your blood test results, your pregnancy scans and information about your baby.

Hair ties: You want your hair out and away from your face so you can breathe properly and cool down. If you are breastfeeding, tie your hair up so you can see the attachment properly. It can also be useful to pop a hair tie on the wrist you last fed from so you don't need to write it down or remember. One less thing to think about.

Face cloth: You will probably get a little hot and sweaty during labour, so not only will this help to cool you down, but if you pop a couple of drops of lavender oil on it, this may also help you feel a little calmer (see page 167 for more on aromatherapy in labour for more details on oils). After you have had your baby it will also come in useful for a nice wash. If you have a Caesarean section you may not be up and walking for a little while, so hospital staff can give you a bed bath with your own cloth or you may prefer to do this yourself.

Birthing ball: I recommend one if you've not got one already. See page 109 for more on the power of the birthing ball.

Snacks and drinks: Although there are snacks in most hospitals you'll want your own favourite foods with you so you don't end up with a sandwich that you don't really fancy. Dark chocolate is a useful energy boost; it's not as sickly or sugary as milk chocolate and it also contains iron, great for both before and after birth. Bring plenty of drinks to keep you hydrated and to keep your sugar levels up – a mix of water and fruit juice is great. Get your partner to pack food for them too – they'll probably be more hungry than you.

Hot water bottle or wheat bag: If you get painful periods you're probably already familiar with this one. Warmth can provide a lovely release and is a real comforter on the lower back/pelvis in labour.

Music: Make a playlist for labour, whether hypnobirthing tracks or pop music. The power of music is phenomenal.

Your own pillow: It makes such a difference to have a bit of home comfort with you.

Something to birth in, and for afterwards: An old nightshirt or long T-shirt is ideal for birthing in (if you're not having a water birth) and take a clean one for afterwards (buttons are useful to make breastfeeding easier). The amount of times I have walked into a room where the baby is crying as mums trying to tuck her pyjama top up under her neck whilst attaching her baby to the breast; it's a real nuisance for them. Instead, go for a super soft and comfy nightshirt that unbuttons down the front so you can feed without hassle of getting your top off or pulling it up and struggling to see. Also (not glamourous) you may want to change your pad whilst standing, especially after a C-section – lifting your nightie saves the day!

Soft slippers: Even if you don't wear them at home usually, take a pair for hygiene and to protect your feet from the hospital floor – go for the non-slip ones.

Toiletries: You'll probably want to have a bath or shower soon after birth. Bring in your regular toiletries and maybe something a little more indulgent like a luxury hair conditioner, even if it's just a sample from an expensive luxury brand. You deserve a little extra.

Sanitary pads: Not just for after but for when/if your waters go. There is a lot of fluid and you'll need plenty of pads. You'll bleed quite heavily after birth – many women are surprised by their blood loss (lochia) – so go for the proper thick maternity pads. If you give birth vaginally you will be more sensitive, so opt for natural, chlorine and bleach-free pads.

Nipple cream: A common reason women stop breastfeeding is because their nipples get too sore. Position and attachment are key and I'll go through what you need to know about breastfeeding on page 285. But caring for breastfeeding nipples is also really helpful. Get a natural nipple cream and use it from the first feed; it really helps to protect and heal your nipples early on. You can also use it as a lip balm in labour, which is great when using gas and air.

Maternity knickers: Go for real Bridget Jones-style big pants because comfort is key after you have had a baby. Make sure they rise right up above your belly button to support your tummy and avoid any potential wounds. TENA disposable pants are a good option.

Breastfeeding: Your breasts will need support after birth, whether you choose to breastfeed or not. Breastfeeding bras are super comfy as they don't have underwire so they don't dig in or pose a risk of you developing mastitis (infection usually caused by blocked ducts). They are easy to feed in, as you can release one cup at a time.

Going home outfit: You might want a change of clothes from the ones you went in with. Stick with your maternity clothes for now as your body will still be adjusting. I suggest a comfy maternity dress. They take up less room in your bag, you don't need to worry about the fit, you haven't got to think about a matching top to go with your bottoms, they are airy and don't rub anywhere that could be sore and they are much easier to get on and off.

GETTING THERE AND BACK!

Have a think about how you plan to get to your place of birth and home again. You will need to have a safe mode of transport for baby with you, such as a car seat. Some hospital guidelines recommend that midwives briefly assess your mode of transport to ensure it's safe before you leave. If possible, it will be more comfortable for you to get a lift or a taxi home because you should avoid walking, even if it is just a ten-minute walk, shortly after giving birth.

YOGA DURING PREGNANCY

~~~

Scientific research has confirmed that meditation, yoga, breathing techniques, walking in nature, forest bathing and visualisation all help us to counteract the stressed state of being that many of us experience in our lives. Pregnancy is a great place to take stock, and think about how you can learn breath control, relaxation and meditation, if you choose.

Feeling stressed is an ancient survival strategy to help us to do the 'fight or flight' thing relating to the threat or perceived threat. A perceived threat, physical or mental, has a stress reaction in the body causing a hormonal release or chemicals (adrenalin and cortisol), which in turn causes the breath and heart rate to increase. If you are feeling anxious during your pregnancy, or just want some time out for relaxation and stretching, yoga can be really helpful.

My mum, Julie, has been practising yoga for over 30 years and is a yoga for pregnancy teacher; she has written this section for the book.

I recommend you go to a yoga class, and try and find one that's yoga for pregnancy. Most teachers advise attending a specialist pregnancy class from 14–15 weeks pregnant, as your pregnancy will be well-established by that time and hopefully you will have stopped feeling the nausea and other symptoms most commonly associated with the first trimester.

In pregnancy, the advice is to go slow and gentle. Of course, there are times when you need to push yourself a little – you will certainly need to find strength and stamina to call on in labour and birth so it is good training. But now that you're pregnant and will be turning inward, it's a time to complement your body and work with it in a gentle, nurturing way. If you nurture yourself, you're nurturing your baby at the same time.

Clearing mental space

As well as learning useful breathing practices, yoga, meditation and other practices can also teach you about 'space'. There's plenty of space for your baby to grow in your body and your organs will just be gently nudged out of the way in the process. It also helps to create some mental space ready for

CHECK WITH YOUR HEALTH PROFESSIONAL

As yoga is so gentle, it's appropriate for most pregnant women, but if you have health issues related to your pregnancy, do check with your midwife or doctor first. Even if you have done lots of yoga before, you might want to join a yoga for pregnancy class, especially if your first pregnancy.

the baby, to clear out old beliefs, unnecessary clutter and stale energy from your mind.

Try this decluttering exercise as much as you feel you need to. As you establish a regular practice, it will become easier to release old hurts, irritations and grudges. You will start to feel generally lighter in yourself and find that you have more headspace.

1. Sit comfortably and quietly, preferably sitting up against a wall with your back straight.
2. Start by closing your eyes and taking a few slow, deep breaths, in and out, until you feel a little more relaxed. Become aware of any mental clutter that you have accumulated such as old hurts, grudges or habitual irritations.
3. Now take your awareness to your out-breath and each time you breathe out, let go … Let go of long-term, stale issues that you've been carrying around for a while now. Those emotional and mental tensions originate outside of you, in the external world. Let it go, breathe out and let go even more.
4. In this moment, allow yourself to feel lighter, relieved of mental clutter and feel the extra space in your head. Allow your brain to feel rested, sitting freely in the skull.
5. Take a moment to relax your neck and throat, let your shoulders drop and feel the weight of any burdens falling away.
6. Enjoy the relaxation. Spend a few minutes sitting or lying, staying with the relaxation and peace, the sense of lightness and space. When you are ready, take your awareness to your breathing again and allow your breath to return to normal.

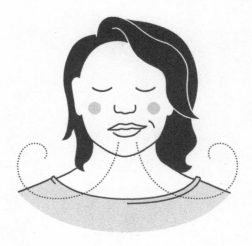

A YOGA BALL

Possibly one of the best investments you will make will be a yoga ball. Women use these to practice pregnancy yoga and during birth classes to try labour positions. A yoga ball is a useful prop for you during labour and can help you to feel more confident and in control. Instead of a yoga ball you can use also use a large bean bag.

Hip circling

Think belly dancing in slow motion! This is an easy yoga movement that will release tension as you move. Stay relaxed and keep the movements smooth and rhythmical.

1. Stand with your legs hip-width apart.
2. Circle your hips clockwise slowly, about five times.
3. Start with a small circle, increasing the size of the circle with practice. Keep your knees soft and slightly bent.
4. Use a wall to support you if you prefer; lean forward, with folded arms onto the wall. Lean your head onto your hands, if you like.
5. Repeat the circles anticlockwise.

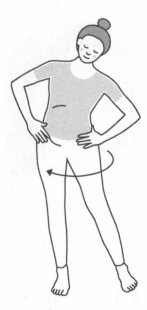

Variation: You can also practise circular motions on your yoga ball, which feels really good in your hips and lower back, and you have the soft support of the ball under your perineum. In labour, this circular movement can be soothing and helpful, so practise it often.

Simple stretches

Lots of women wonder if it's okay to exercise during pregnancy. The answer is almost always an emphatic yes! Gentle stretching is possible right through your pregnancy and will help to keep you supple and mobile for labour. Stretching during pregnancy can also feel great and can help to release some of the tension you feel from carrying a small person around inside you!

1. Stand next to a table or kitchen worktop and place your hands on it, about shoulder-width apart. Lean forward gently until you can feel a gentle stretch in your lower back.
2. You could also try this sitting on your yoga ball, facing the wall and stretching your arms up the wall.
3. In either position, now shrug and circle your shoulders a few times to release any tension there.
4. Now take your arms behind you to stretch the arms, shoulders and front of your chest.

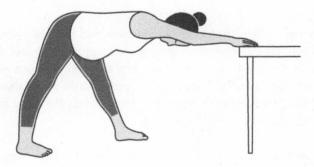

Hip opener

As your pregnancy progresses, you can help your hips to open and stretch ready for labour. Making space for your baby is one of your goals and these postures will help.

1. Sit with your legs crossed gently at the ankles. Use cushions to pop under your knees if necessary.
2. Now bring the soles of your feet together and let your knees fall apart. The further away you take your feet from your bottom, the less strenuous this posture will feel.
3. If comfortable, make small 'butterfly wing' movements, bringing your knees gently up and down. Then stop, and allow the weight of your knees and gravity to drop your knees lower, without any force or strain. The more you work with gravity and relax, the easier it becomes.
4. Do these movements in sync with the breath. Breathe in as your knees fall away and out as you bring them back together. Spend a few minutes doing this on a daily basis.

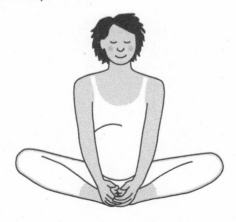

Squats

Gentle, supported squats are good hip openers and help to prepare you for labour positions. Your perineum is able to relax in a squat too. Check with your midwife in the third trimester if you are okay to continue with squats, depending on baby's position; deep squats are not advisable after 34 weeks. Also anyone with haemorrhoids won't be doing themselves any favours with deep squats as this could make them worse.

1. With a partner opposite, hold each other by the wrists. Stand with your legs hip-width apart and slowly and carefully squat down until you feel that's enough – you need to communicate well with your partner.
2. As you lower, make sure your bottom is moving back (like you are going to sit on a chair). Check that your knees are always going in the same direction as your feet. You can choose to have your feet pointing forwards or slightly out to the side but to protect your knees, always have them going in the same direction as your feet. Use the outbreath as you gently squat down and breathe in as you return to standing. Don't hold squats for too long; try to keep them dynamic (moving), coming up and down smoothly, slowly and gently.
3. If you want to squat on your own, try using your yoga ball between your back and the wall and rock or squat gently. Breathe out as you lower and in as you come back up.
4. Aim for just a few squats at a time, using them to build up strength in your legs and getting used to how low you want to go.

Preparing your perineum

THIS SECTION COVERS most women's biggest fear: tearing. This section isn't the most glamorous of all, so let's get all the vocab out there that we need to use: anus, vagina, tearing, floppy fanny, ring of fire, rectum, down there ... Midwives have heard it all, so don't be shy to use whatever vocab you want when talking to us about your body.

The perineum is the small area of firm skin and muscular tissue between your vagina and anus and this where your body makes room for your baby. Something that most women are worried about is tearing the perineum and surrounding area. Don't worry, we are going to go through everything that you can do to help prevent this from happening.

YOUR AMAZING VAGINA

Ever seen a penis significantly change shape and size? It is not just penises that can do this; your vagina and perineum have this amazing changing ability too. Vaginas are especially designed to stretch and change shape as your baby's head comes down through your pelvis. I remember the first few times I saw this happen as a student and being really surprised at how well the vagina and perineum can stretch and open – I had no idea it could do this so well.

Relaxing and opening
Your perineum needs to relax so it can stretch, open properly and perform at its best. If you are squeezing your muscles in any way, then your body isn't able to stretch in the way that it is designed to. Opening and tensing do not

121

work well together, and usually tensing wins the battle if you don't know how to relax. Practising how to relax your entire pelvic floor will give you better results in labour, so here's how:

The muscles you would use to stop yourself from peeing are the muscles you need to relax. Try giving them a squeeze now ... and relax. Fully allow everything to drop down, including your abdominal muscles. Notice how there is no tension, holding or squeezing – you're lower half is fully relaxed – this is exactly what you want during birth. You will find that relaxing your mouth and jaw helps this too. Let your jaw hang down slightly and move it from side to side, open up a little wider and now fully yawn. You may hear some little cracks or pops; that's good – we hold a lot of tension in our jaw. Now let your jaw relax and hang down again. You may notice it feels that little bit softer, more spacious and easily open. These simple and easy exercises can help to release and relax your perineum too. As internationally known midwife Ina May Gaskin says: 'floppy face, floppy fanny.'

MASSAGE YOUR PERINEUM

~~~~~

The other thing that has been proven to really help is perineal massage, because massage helps the connective tissues become as supple and elastic as possible. This is ancient stuff and women have been doing it globally for generations, but it has only fairly recently become popular in the UK. Research tells us that perineal massage is most successful for first-time mums. If you have a vaginal infection or herpes it's best to avoid but check with your midwife as there are exceptions. Also make sure your nails aren't too long or pointed in shape.

Around 34 weeks is a good time to start massaging, and it is best to do it after a nice warm bath or shower, when your blood vessels are dilated. Being relaxed and warm makes the perineum a bit softer and more comfortable to touch. The kindest massage oils to use are unscented and organic, like olive oil or grapeseed oil. Avoid oils with chemicals in.

1. Get into a comfortable position; there are lots of positions to try. Try either sitting up with a pillow propped up behind you in bed, on all-fours, or in the bath, shower or on the toilet, whatever works best for you. Some

women ask their partners to do this for them but most women prefer to do it themselves. It doesn't really matter who does it, just that it's done properly and you are able to relax throughout.

2. Put one or both of your thumbs a few centimetres inside your vagina in the centre, towards the back wall. Relax your other fingers onto your bum cheeks.

PERINEAL MASSAGE

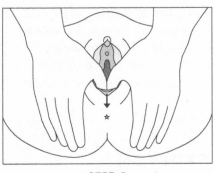

STEP 2

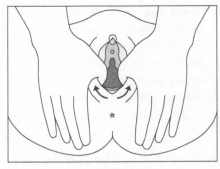

STEP 5

3. Press down with your thumbs towards your rectum and then sideways as you breathe out and fully relax your lower jaw and mouth like we practised a minute ago.

4. Hold your thumbs in this position for one to two minutes and continue to breathe. You will begin to feel a slight burning or stretching sensation. It should not be painful.

5. Then massage up and out creating a U-shape, sweeping like motion. Your aim here is to massage the inside area of your vagina, not just the skin on the outside. You'll probably feel the skin stretching on the outside but you want to get focused on the massaging and stretching inside. This is similar to the sensation you'll get as your baby is being born.

6. Relax your perineum as much as possible to get the most out of your massage, keep breathing and keep your facial muscles relaxed. It shouldn't hurt and you do need to be gentle too. Remember how stretching and tensing don't work together.

7. Wash your hands afterwards.

Tip: After you have been massaging at least twice a week, you'll get the hang of it and gradually be able to increase the pressure. Your perineum will start to become more elastic. By practising this at the end of pregnancy you'll have more control during labour and are less likely to tense up when you start to feel the familiar pressure. Try to implement it into your morning or bedtime routine so you don't forget.

There are products on the market that claim to reduce tears and episiotomies, but as far as I am aware, there's not enough credible research to support these claims. It is probably best to get to know your perineum yourself, apply your own pressure and use your own hands. If you don't already know your vagina and perineum well, it is a good idea to get to know them in pregnancy.

WARM AND STRETCH

Warm compresses placed on the perineum have been used by midwives with great success over the years. Hannah Dahlen (a midwifery legend) was a student midwife in the UK, and she remembers seeing a woman in labour who, although close to giving birth, seemed scared of letting her baby come out. The supervising midwife (with a lot of experience) quietly got up, left the room, and returned a few minutes later with a bowl of warm water. She put a cloth in the water, wrung it out, and placed it gently on the woman's perineum. The woman's face relaxed noticeably, and she gave birth to her baby. When questioned about what the water was for, the senior midwife answered, 'Just soothing the ring of fire, ducky.'

Hannah went on to undertake the largest trial, now known as the warm pack trial. The results showed that warm compresses applied to the perineum during the second stage of labour (when you are pushing and your baby's head is visible) *halved* the rate of severe perineal trauma by helping the perineum to relax and open, as well as helping with comfort during the birth and the first couple of days afterwards. Her study also found bladder control was far better three months following the birth. So many wins for such a simple thing. Thanks to Hannah and her colleagues, perineal warm packs are now accepted as an approved technique to reduce perineal trauma. Most midwives do know about this but it is worth putting a note in your birth plan to be sure; you don't need to pack your own flannel as we have sterile pads that we can use in our birth packs.

The vaginal muscles and tissue are easily able to stretch when given the best opportunity to, and right environment. You are giving your perineum the best opportunity by working with your body, learning to relax, doing perineal massage in pregnancy, and by keeping it warm in labour. All of these make natural birth that little bit easier.

IF TEARING HAPPENS

Tearing is more common with first babies and a lot of women don't even know they have had one. Some won't need stitching, because your vagina also has this amazing ability to self-heal. I have seen lots perineums heal beautifully all by themselves. If you have a tear that is bleeding or is a little deeper, stitches may be recommend. You'll be offered pain relief for this and depending on the nature of the tear, either a doctor (usually in theatre) or a midwife can do this for you. For more on postnatal/perineal healing see page 256.

KEY POINTS

- Antenatal yoga classes can help to prepare your body for birth, and calm the mind. You can also meet lots of other pregnant women.
- Your vagina is designed to stretch and open.
- Work with your vagina's natural abilities by letting go and relaxing down below.
- Relax your jaw and mouth to relax your perineum.
- Massage your perineum from 34 weeks.
- Ask for a warm compress during the second stage of labour.

PELVIC FLOOR EXERCISES

~~~~

Your pelvic floor is a powerful set of muscles, ligaments and fibrous tissue. They look a bit like a hammock and sit between your tailbone and public bone. Your pelvic floor is a big deal because it plays an important role in core stability, bladder and bowel control and sexual function. Pelvic floor problems affect up to 80 per cent of expectant and new mums.

The pelvic floor is under a lot of strain in pregnancy but the good news is you can strengthen the muscles by doing pelvic floor exercises now. Doing these in pregnancy helps to reduce and avoid stress incontinence after you have had your baby. In an ideal world, all pregnant women would do pelvic floor exercises, even if you're young and don't have stress incontinence now (leaking wee when you cough or sneeze).

Physiotherapist Lizzie Kellaway has got some good advice and easy home exercises you can do to help regain strength in your pelvic floor to prevent incontinence and prolapse later on in life. Here is what she has to say about looking after your pelvic floor:

'In pregnancy the pelvic floor muscles are under increasing pressure to support the growing baby. Often in the later stages of pregnancy you may start to feel the strain on the pelvic floor muscles. For example, inability to hold on when you need to get to the loo or having a surprise leak. Postnatally, if these symptoms start to occur or increase then it's highly likely that your pelvic floor has lost some strength.

'It is important to take care of the pelvic floor muscles after childbirth (see page 258), no matter if it was a Caesarean section or a vaginal delivery. The best way to do this is to exercise the muscles and allow them time to heal effectively.

'Sometimes, with larger perineal tears, bladder and bowel symptoms may be more severe, and vaginal or perineal scarring can be uncomfortable, particularly with sex. If this is the case it is important to see a women's health physiotherapist at around six weeks postnatally.

'If possible, try to get some help with strenuous activities and try to sit down before lifting heavy objects or holding children.

'**Note:** Running is not advised before three months postnatally, or beyond this if any symptoms of pelvic floor problems such as incontinence or prolapse are identified.'

How to do pelvic floor exercises

The good news is you can do your pelvic floor exercises anywhere, at any time! Just do not do them whilst you are weeing. Initially it may be easier to do them lying down and you can then try them sitting, or standing. Aim to do these twice a day, not just postnatally but forever and always!

1. Pull up your muscles from your back passage as if you are stopping yourself from passing wind and weeing. Try not to hold your breath. Squeeze your bottom muscles, inner thigh muscles and draw in your stomach muscles tightly.
2. See if you can hold your muscles for up to ten seconds and notice when the muscles let themselves relax. Keep to this length of holding until you can hold for longer.
3. Try and do some quick contractions and see how many you can do, up to ten times.

THE PELVIC FLOOR:

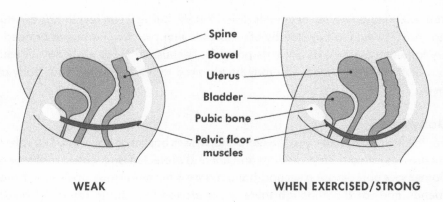

Spine
Bowel
Uterus
Bladder
Pubic bone
Pelvic floor muscles

WEAK   WHEN EXERCISED/STRONG

Creating a nest

NOW YOU KNOW how to plan and pack for birth, it is a good time to have a think about creating your nest at home, ready for baby to arrive.

Parents sometimes worry about money and not being able to afford the latest products, clothes and toys for their baby. They sometimes worry about what other people think and their social status. Your baby doesn't care about social status, what car you drive, who you've just impressed or whether or not they are wearing 'hand-me-downs'. All that matters to them is you. Your touch, your skin, your smell and your voice.

Don't worry if you can't afford the latest stuff; you are enough.

You will need a few key essentials (listed below) but you can buy things as you go. You'll be told to buy stuff by other people that you may never use or need. Try to keep your nest as basic as possible, because in those early days if you buy stuff you don't need, you may be too tired to return it when your baby is here.

Baby's bed

For the first few months, you'll need a crib, Moses basket or travel cot. The safest mattresses for your baby are firm and flat and protected by a waterproof cover. Sometimes parents use a second-hand mattress from previous children or from friends and family. Although there is no proven link, some research shows an increased chance of SIDS (Sudden Infant Death Syndrome) when using a second-hand mattress brought in from outside of the family home. Generally, it is safest to have a new mattress for each baby but if this is not possible make sure the mattress was previously completely protected by a waterproof cover, with no rips or tears and is in good condition. The mattress should also still be firm and flat to keep your baby safe while sleeping. Your baby needs to sleep close by to you, somewhere that is safe and warm. They won't need any pillows and duvets because they're not safe until your baby is a year old. As well as potentially covering your baby's face, duvets can also make your baby too hot, which is particularly dangerous for newborns. A baby sleeping bag is a good option for keeping your baby warm and is recommended by the Lullaby Trust – ensure you get the right tog and size. Sheets or blankets are also fine but it is really important that you tuck them in firmly *below* your baby's shoulder level and put your baby 'feet to foot', with their feet right at the end

CO-SLEEPING

The best advice is to ensure your baby has a clear space to sleep in your room but in their own Moses basket or cot. Although I do not recommend co-sleeping, it is important to recognise that many parents do co-sleep. Stats show that it is on the increase in the UK and co-sleeping is also the norm for a very high percentage of the world's population, so we need to cover it here to ensure that should you choose to co-sleep, you do so safely.

- Do not share a bed with your baby if you or your partner smoke or have drunk alcohol or taken drugs – including prescription drugs.
- The safest kind of co-sleeping is planned. Keep pillows, sheets and blankets away from your baby or any other items that could obstruct your baby's breathing or cause them to overheat.
- Make sure your baby is flat on their back and that your mattress is firm, flat and waterproof.
- Make sure your baby can't fall out of bed or get trapped between the mattress and the wall.
- Do not leave the baby alone in the bed to sleep.
- Avoid letting pets or other children in the bed.
- Do not co-sleep on a sofa or armchair – this can significantly increase the risk of SIDS.

of the crib, basket or cot, so that they can't wriggle down under the covers. For more on choosing safe bedding see www.lullabytrust.org.uk/safer-sleep-advice/sleeping-products.

Room thermometer

For any room that your baby is sleeping in (whether bedroom or sitting room) the room temp should be 16–20° Celsius. You may also want to get a thermometer to measure your baby's body temperature too.

Changing mat

These usually come with baby-changing bags if you decide to buy one – if not you can pick up a home baby-changing mat or cot top changer. If you are using the same changing mat out and about and at home, ensure that you clean it properly and wipe down both sides properly after each change.

GETTING OUT AND ABOUT

Once you have created your home nest you need to think about leaving it and how you'll get out and about with your little one. Again there are so many products on the market – it is one that is ever-evolving – so for now we will focus on the key things most new parents need and use regularly.

Car seat

A car seat is essential for travelling in a car or taxi with your baby. If possible, have an adult in the back with your baby, especially in the early weeks when they are more likely to slump down. If not possible, get a clip-on rear-view mirror so you can keep an eye on your baby. Some car seats flatten down slightly and these can be good for longer journeys because you really want to avoid having a small baby slumped over. When buying a car seat look for the United Nations ECE Regulation number R44.03 or R44.04, or the new i-size regulation R129. For more information check out www.childcarseats.org.uk. NHS online have some simple and easy advice.

Pushchairs and prams

Pushchairs (strollers and buggies), are only suitable for young babies if they have fully reclining seats so your baby can lie flat. Wait until your baby can sit by themselves before using another type of pushchair. Go for a light pushchair if you'll be lifting it on to trains or buses.

Prams give your baby a lot of space to sit and lie comfortably, but they take up a lot of space and are hard to use on public transport. If you have a car, look for a pram that can be dismantled easily. Consider buying a pram harness at the same time, as you may need it to strap your baby securely into the pram.

Carrycot/travel system

A carrycot is a light, portable cot with handles, similar to but smaller than the body of a pram, and often attachable to a wheeled frame. Your baby can sleep in the carrycot for the first few months, and the cot can be attached to the frame to go out.

Slings and carriers

Baby-wearing is ancient and practised in many cultures around the world. Babies absolutely love being carried close to you as they feel all safe and warm. They can see what is going on around them in the comfort of your security. They have become super-popular recently and mums and dads say how much easier it is to carry a baby this way. You are hands-free and this makes life easier and more practical. However, if not used correctly, a carrier or sling can be dangerous. Babies are less able to maintain their airway, so remember these safety points if you opt for baby wearing:

- Baby should be held tight to you so they can't fall out.
- Baby's face should be in view at all times.
- Close enough to kiss.
- Keep them in an upright position, with their chin off their chest (the neck shouldn't be able to bend over).
- Baby should have a supported back, and not be able to slump, which can lead to breathing problems.

DISABILITIES AND BECOMING A PARENT

Navigating pregnancy and parenthood with a disability can be tough at times, although I have looked after many women with various disabilities who have found motherhood more empowering than anything before – their trust and respect for their body has never been so great. I wanted to make sure that those of you who have a disability get some extra first-hand advice. I spoke to Ashley Taylor, the founder of disabledparents. org to get her top tips.

Ashley says: 'While there is no way to be completely ready for the parenting experience, planning and preparation can make a big difference in how quickly you adjust to parenthood. If you also have a disability, it's vital to take the necessary steps to ensure a safe and enriching experience. Here are five ways to plan and prepare when you have a disability and are expecting:'

Get the right equipment
First, you want to plan out what equipment you will need. Some of it you will need before your baby arrives, and some of it can wait until later. Also, some conventional items will come ready to use, but if you have a physical disability, you may need to order a speciality product or make some modifications to a product when you get it. Look for items that can make everyday parenting tasks more accessible, such as a breastfeeding sling, side-opening bassinet, adaptive stroller, or a swivel-base car seat.

Modify your home
Along with purchasing specialised equipment, you may need to make some home modifications. The key is to make your home safe and

accessible for your everyday needs. For instance, if you have limited mobility and/or use an aid (wheelchair, walker, etc.), you may need to remove any loose carpet and rugs, and install slip-resistant flooring and mats for when moving around with baby. Also, modifying your sinks, taps and cabinets can make daily tasks easier. Is there space for everything you need? What can you get rid of now, and will you be able to reach everything you need easily?

Look into resources

There are grants and support services specifically for parents with disabilities. Researching and applying for assistance is not always a quick and easy process, so you might want to start this now, rather than after baby is born.

Get help when you need it

Do you need help installing threshold ramps or putting expandable hinges on your doors? Ask for help. Do you need to take a few hours for personal time? Ask someone to watch your little one. If you have people in your life who are willing to help you with the parenting process, please do ask and look on the website for more ideas.

Love more, worry less

Being a new parent can be nerve-racking. It's easy to worry about how you do every little task when it comes to caring for your baby. You want to be the best parent possible and make sure your baby is safe, comfortable and thriving. But if you focus more on simply being present and loving your child, your moments together will be richer, and the details of how to care for them will naturally come as you learn their patterns and needs.

Building a village

FRIENDSHIP IS A universal feature of nearly all human societies – we all need friends. In many cultures and ancient traditions, older women of the village, mothers and aunts, pass down wisdom and look after pregnant women and new mothers. When I lived in Australia, I learnt about pregnancy care and rituals for Aboriginals. Traditionally, they take more of a holistic view of wellbeing, with a supportive extended family network, connection to country, and active cultural practices. Many places around the world still have this approach to birth and new motherhood. We tend not to live like this in the Western world as much any more, and many of us live miles away from the women in our families. Of course, there are some real benefits from moving out of your home town, like having the opportunity to progress in your career and learn or grow as a person, but this can be a disadvantage when raising a baby. It still 'takes a village to raise a child', as the saying goes, no matter where you are or what you do for a job. If you live far away from supportive family, you need to create your own village. Whether they're related or total strangers, most mums share the same worries and hurdles, so if you are usually a little bit shy around new people remember that there will be more things that unite you than divide you as mums. The bonds and pearls of wisdom that you get from other mums or women who understand what you are experiencing is irreplaceable.

'I felt lonely the first time round and I honestly don't know what I'd do without my NCT clan. Three years on we are all still texting nearly every day (more than half are on round two babies!) and we have a shared birthday party every year. We've even picked up each other's kids from nursery when we've been stuck in traffic, we've been to scans and appointments with each other, and we all know everything about each other because of asking for advice about mastitis, chapped nipples, stitches etc. We've been for nights out and are planning a spa session soon. Without my family around they've been my saving grace and I don't know what I'd have done without them. At the beginning some of them did have family around though, and I had to say that I was feeling a bit lonely and asked for invitations to stuff ... which was a bit hard but I'm glad I did as the more they understood my situation, the better it got.'

Shelley, first-time mum

WAYS TO BUILD YOUR VILLAGE

If you want to get out and find your squad, then here are a few options. There will be like-minded people out there, promise.

- Join a yoga for pregnancy class.
- Go to group antenatal classes or hypnobirthing classes. Hypnobirthing classes start at around 25 weeks. You can go with your partner or birth partner too (see page 182 for more on hypnobirthing).
- Look into Positive Birth Movement founded by Millie Hill – they are free to attend antenatal discussion groups, and they're available all around the world.
- Digital antenatal education is an option if you can't or aren't keen on groups – join their online community instead and aim to meet up in person.
- Join free apps like Mums Anywhere, Mush Mums or Peanut.
- Join Facebook groups like 'Top Tips 4 Mums' or 'Channel Mum'.
- If you are planning on breastfeeding, research local support groups now.
- Talk to other pregnant women you meet – smile and say hello. After all, you've got something majorly obvious in common.

GOING TO ANTENATAL CLASSES

Even if you have read all the books and have spoken to your midwife at length, I think it is worth going to antenatal classes to build confidence in your knowledge and to meet other women at your stage of pregnancy. There are many private classes available, as well as classes organised and covered by your local hospital. It is best to start antenatal classes when you're well into your third trimester, around 32 weeks.

'As midwives, we want women to be active participants in their care – to know the choices they have available to them, and to be able to make confident, informed decisions throughout their pregnancy, labour and beyond. Antenatal education, in some form, is imperative to achieve this. Whether it's a group course, a one-to-one session, an online tutorial, or reading endless books, antenatal preparation is key to achieving a better birth experience.'

Katie and Leila, founders of Better Births Antenatal Classes

'Before the class we had some understanding about labour as we had done a hypnobirthing class, however, there was still a lot we didn't know.

'The class was broken down really clearly and the techniques and games used to teach us were great and really made you remember things. There were a lot of visuals and clear explanations which all helped the learning process.

'My husband also learned a lot as he knew less than me on labour and baby care, and he found it really useful and interesting.'

Siobhan and Craig, first-time parents

Zwischen – the last few days of pregnancy

UNLESS YOU SPEAK German you probably wouldn't have heard the word 'Zwischen' before. It means 'in between' and a midwife called Jana Studelska thought it was about time that we had a name for those last few days of pregnancy, quite rightly so – 'Zwischen' it is. Jana refers to this time as 'Neither here nor there. Your old self and your new self, balanced on the edge of a pregnancy. One foot in your old world, one foot in a new world. I believe that this is more than biological. It is spiritual, a woman must go to the place between this world and the next ... she is going to the edge of her being where every resource she has will be called on to assist in this journey.'

One of the most distinctive times during pregnancy is sort of abandoned and seen as just the waiting time. When we wait for anything in life, the longer we wait the more we start to feel a sense of urgency creeping in. To increase this sense of urgency, women then start to feel the pressure to go into labour from both friends/family and professionals – this can really taint the end of your epic journey to motherhood. You should be feeling, calm, confident and relaxed to give your body the best chance of going into labour naturally. So that is what this section is about, we are going to explore this abandoned time, think about a few things you can do with the time and also run over why your due date should (almost) be ignored.

WHAT TO DO DURING ZWISCHEN

This is a very special time in your life. You may only ever truly experience it once in your entire life (that is) often before the birth of your first baby. You've got everything ready, your body and life have dramatically changed and you start to feel like a mum but ... you're still pregnant. Maybe your 'due date' has come and gone and you're left waiting and wondering in anticipation.

The good news is that there are things you can be doing in this time. Try to enjoy the extra day or two (or seven or more ...) and do things that you may not have time to do once your baby has arrived. I always tell mums to have things planned past their due date so you have something nice to look forward to. Here's a suggested list:

- Book reflexology (for pregnancy) or a facial.
- List a few funny films or box sets you want to watch but haven't got around to.
- Catch up with your mum, sister or bestie for a morning coffee or lunch.
- Have a calming, candle-lit lavender bath.
- Have a date/chill night with your partner/birth partner, in or out – whatever you prefer.
- Read a light-hearted book you've been meaning to read.
- Go shopping for three (cheap) dressing gowns – it makes such a difference to have a change of gown if you don't leave the house for a week after birth (see below).
- Cook and freeze meals to refuel your postnatal body if you feel like it.
- Listen to some funny podcasts or watch funny YouTube clips. Even though this time is abandoned, try not to abandon your sense of humour. Laughing and smiling release happy hormones making you feel more at ease.

DRESSED FOR THE OCCASION

The three dressing gowns are for after you have had your baby. It is normal to not get dressed properly and be in your dressing gown for most of the day. It is also normal to not want to leave the house for a week or two. If you rotate your dressing gowns it makes it feel more acceptable – kind of like you have a different outfit every couple of days. Your temperature will also fluctuate with hormonal changes, some women get bad night sweats, so if you have a few that are different materials that can help. Plus, at least one is most likely going to end up with baby sick, food or some sort of stain down it; if you're dressed for the occasion it doesn't matter.

FOOD GLORIOUS FOOD

Making food shouldn't be a job for you as a new mum so, if you feel like it, use your time before baby arrives to cook some healthy hearty meals and freeze them (or pass this section on to your partner!). Many cultures believe that warming foods and broths promote healing and prevent postnatal depletion; slow-cooked, warming food like chicken or vegetable soups and stews are ideal. In some cultures, new mothers won't eat *anything* cold for at least 40 days after birth. Soups, broths and stews are cheap, easy to make, and freeze really well. Laura Hughes (see page 51) has a couple of recipes here for you to prep ahead of time.

LAMB AND MANGO COCONUT CURRY

Lamb contains lots of B vitamins and zinc to help deal with anxiety and stress, both common side effects of motherhood! This curry is a nutritional powerhouse full of iron to help with fatigue, and other nutrients to help support the body at times of repair and nutrient depletion. Micronutrients (vitamins and minerals) are essential for us to turn our macronutrients, such as carbohydrates, into useable energy. This is a mild curry so add more spice if you like, and double-up as you like to put some in the freezer.

SERVES 2

400g organic diced lamb
1 tbsp ground turmeric
2 tbsp mild curry powder

1 tbsp garam masala
1 white onion, diced

1 thumb-sized piece of root ginger, grated
400g can full-fat coconut milk
1 garlic clove, crushed
400g can chopped tomatoes
1 fresh mango, sliced

2 tbsp mango chutney
100g almond flour
1 handful spinach (can use chard or kale if preferred)
Olive oil, for cooking

TO SERVE
Brown rice, sesame seeds, freshly chopped coriander, lime

Place the lamb in a large casserole pan with a glug of olive oil, along with the turmeric, curry powder, garam masala, onion and ginger. Cook on a medium heat for about 3 minutes until the meat has turned golden brown. Now add the coconut milk, garlic and the canned tomatoes and leave to simmer on the lowest heat on your hob for about 10 minutes.

Meanwhile, pop your rice on to cook as per the cooking instructions. When the rice is nearing its cooking time, add the mango slices, mango chutney, almond flour and spinach to the curry mix. Stir through and leave to simmer until the rice is ready.

Serve the rice and curry with a sprinkling of sesame seeds, coriander and a squeeze of lime.

MAKE IT VEGAN: Swap the lamb for chickpeas, lentils or tofu. If using tofu, add towards the end of cooking time with the mango slices.

SUPER HEALING SOUP

This soothing soup contains collagen for repair of tissues, prebiotics for gut health, protein for healing and fibre for good digestion.

SERVES 2

1 butternut squash, (about 1kg), peeled and cut into 2cm chunks
6 tbsp olive oil
8 unpeeled garlic cloves
1 tbsp apple cider vinegar

½ tsp paprika
2 leeks, roughly chopped
2 celery stalks, chopped into 1cm cubes
1 red chilli, thinly sliced

400g can butterbeans, rinsed and drained

3 rosemary sprigs

1 litre chicken bone broth or vegetable stock

1 tbsp pumpkin seeds

3 tbsp coconut yoghurt

Salt and pepper, to taste

Bread, to serve, if you like

Preheat the oven to 200°C/400°F. Place the butternut squash cubes, 3 tbsp of the olive oil, the garlic, vinegar and paprika in a roasting tin and mix together. Cook for 20 minutes, take out and turn, then place back in the oven for another 20 minutes.

Meanwhile, put the remaining olive oil, leeks and celery in a large saucepan, and cook on a low heat for around 15 minutes until softened. Add the chilli, butterbeans and rosemary sprigs, stir and cook for a further few minutes.

Remove the butternut squash from the oven and add to the pan with the chicken bone broth or vegetable stock and 500ml of cold water. Bring to the boil, then reduce the heat and let it simmer for 20 minutes.

Meanwhile, quickly toast the pumpkin seeds in a frying pan until golden brown.

Remove the soup from the hob, and de-stalk the rosemary leaving just the leaves in the pan. Add the coconut yoghurt and blend the soup with a blender.

Serve in soup bowls with the seeds sprinkled on top.

LOOKING AFTER YOUR MIND

~~~

As well as looking after your body, with nourishing food, do take care of your mind too. I am a big fan of keeping a hand-written log or journal of how you are feeling, with your thoughts, fears, frustrations and emotions. It is good to get them out of your head and onto paper. No one else needs to read them but it is healthy for you to recognise what is going on in your mind at this time. You may also forget, once your baby is here, what life was like before you became a mum and it can be insightful to look back at the person you are right now.

You could try morning and evening visualisations too. Sit on a birthing ball or chair with your hips open. Imagine ('visualise') your body softening and opening. Very gently stretch from side to side, and open your arms out fully (like Rose on *Titanic* – it's liberating!). Repeat out loud, or in your mind: 'I am ready, I am open and I trust my body.' Relax your arms then imagine holding your baby for the first time, exploring their little face, think about how soft their skin is. Vividly picture their little hands, toes and eyelashes. You will soon be doing this for real and thinking about it now can help you mentally prepare.

LET IT ALL OUT!

Cry when you feel like it. Lots of women hold back the tears because they don't know why they feel like crying, so they think they shouldn't, or they feel silly. You have been through so much and you are right up at the end of your journey, on the cusp of motherhood. It is normal to feel emotional about this, so try to avoid pushing your feelings away. It is totally fine to sit and have a sob on your own, with your birth partner, with a pal or with your midwife. Sometimes this wave of emotion can be the start of a pre-labour clear out; your body could be creating space emotionally and physically. This wave can be caused by pregnancy hormones and the transition your body needs to go through to go into labour. Wherever the feeling is coming from, let it all out. It's okay.

You may end up doing both of these exercises, or none of the above; either way it does not matter. Your state of mind is what matters most at this time.

HOW LONG IS PREGNANCY MEANT TO BE?

Let's get straight to the point and answer this question directly: there is no known exact length of pregnancy. Your due date is an estimation. Just 3–5 per cent of babies arrive on their due date and around 80–85 per cent of first time mums go 'overdue'. A body that has never given birth before may just need a little more time; think about it from your body's perspective. Your body has spent the entire pregnancy protecting, growing and literally holding your baby inside, with an impressive array of defence mechanisms to prevent pre-term birth. Then it needs to completely change track, ditch the Braxton Hicks rehearsals and go for it!

Midwives and doctors base your first estimated due date (EDD) on your last menstrual period (LMP). At the 12 weeks 'dating scan', the final estimated due date is generally decided. Notice the word 'estimated'.

In the UK, a full-term pregnancy is considered to be anything from 37 weeks up to 42 weeks, although an induction is generally recommended at 41+5 to aim for birth by 42 weeks. This four- to five-week period is considered to be a 'window of normality' because it is well understood that the due date is just an estimation. Not much in human existence is standard. We all get hungry at different times and we grow hair at different rates. Given how different we are how strange would it be if all pregnancies were exactly the same length and all babies were born at 40 weeks? We expect a baby to come anywhere within that time frame but not necessarily on a given day. Globally, we don't agree on the normal length of pregnancy either. In the UK we say 40 weeks, in France it's 41 weeks, and in some parts of the world no one expects anything until 42 weeks.

An interesting paper, *'Length of human pregnancy and contributors to its natural variation,'* published in 2013, found there is a wide variation of pregnancy length. It concludes:

'The length of human gestation varies considerably among healthy pregnancies, even when ovulation is accurately measured. This variability is greater than suggested by the clinical assignment of a single "due date". The duration of previous pregnancies may provide a useful measure of a woman's "natural" length of pregnancy and may help in predicting an individual woman's due date.'

We are used to having timely expectations. We track our parcels, can watch our taxis approach us through an app, and get same-day delivery. Natural birth does not fall into our modern-day expectations of punctuality, and if you're aiming for a natural birth, the best thing you can do is accept this fully. You can almost ignore your due date and expect your baby to come a little after it.

> ### 'The trick is to enjoy life. Don't wish away your days, waiting for better ones ahead.'
>
> — **MARJORIE PAY HINCKLEY**

Accepting this date flexibility can be easier for you than it is for everyone else. I have had many women break down in tears during their routine antenatal appointment after going overdue; not only because they had their own expectations, but because every single person that has their number won't stop asking, 'Have you had the baby yet?!'

So, how do you get around this? You could tell people how many weeks you are, then let them try to figure it out. You could tell people, 'It's a spring baby' or if they push for a specific date say, 'Due around April time.' If you just want to fob them off all together, say the date that's two weeks *after* your EDD. If you have already told people your due date you can tell them it got changed and you're now due two weeks later. That way you won't get bombarded with 'Still pregnant?', or 'I bet you are fed up now' and my personal favourite, 'Aren't they doing anything about that?!'

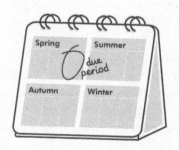

INDUCTION OF LABOUR

~~~~

In the NHS, an induction of labour is generally offered at 41 weeks +5 days. (National Institute for Health and Care Excellence) NICE recommend women should 'be offered induction of labour between 41 weeks +0 and 42 weeks +0 to avoid the risks of prolonged pregnancy. The exact timing should take into account the woman's preferences and local circumstances'. But your midwife may well ask if she should book your induction 'just in case', about a week before then. Agreeing to have the induction booked may feel like you now have added 'pressure to perform', as some women have told me. That is not a nice feeling, I know. Firstly, remember that you do not have to book anything in advance if you do not want to; simply saying 'no thanks' and giving it a couple of days is up to you. Secondly, the main reason your midwife is suggesting you book in advance is mostly for the hospital's planning and logistics. In order to ensure that everyone gets the best care possible, managers need to plan staffing levels, skill mix and each individual women's needs. Our processing and planning can make you feel like your midwife is expecting you to go overdue or losing faith in your ability. She isn't, I promise: she is just making sure that you have an appointment available should you want or need it. You can also change your mind at any time. Have it booked in and then decide you'd rather not on the day, if you like – that is completely fine.

NICE guidelines also state: 'Although the risks of fetal compromise and stillbirth rise steeply after 42 weeks, this rise is from a low baseline. Consequently, only a comparatively small proportion of that population is at particular risk. Because there is no way to precisely identify those pregnancies, delivery currently has to be recommended to all such women. If there were better methods of predicting complications in an individual pregnancy, induction of labour could be more precisely directed towards those at particular risk.'

The topic of induction for going overdue is heavily debated. One of the thoughts behind recommending induction is due to the question over the ability of the placenta to continue to perform as well as it has been (known as 'placental insufficiency') and the rise in adverse outcome after 42 weeks. The data available about placental maturity and sufficiency is complex but also scarce. The bottom line is there is a mix of expert opinion and evidence around the world, and it is down to individual circumstances and background.

Guidelines are there to help guide best practice, but not everyone fits into one guideline. For example, according to a 2008 study including 442,596 women, more South Asian and black women appear to give birth before 39 weeks and their babies appear to be more developed at this time than those of white women.

If an induction is recommended, and you think that you would like to wait a little longer, then you should ask your midwife about your *personal* risks of doing this. You can also ask about any other options to keep an eye on how your baby is doing. For example, can you have additional monitoring like CTGs or an extra scan to check the blood flow to your baby? You also need to think about other risks factors. For example, have you had any need for additional scans in pregnancy already, or have you developed any complications? Have you been happy with your baby's movement over the past few weeks? What else is happening? All of these are little pieces to the puzzle that give a better picture of your baby's wellbeing, and lead to a decision that is best for you and your baby. Those considerations are not exhaustive or conclusive; they are just things to get you thinking about looking at the whole picture (see page 37, BRAIN).

KEY POINTS

- Relax, eat and organise some meals for after you've had your baby.
- A very small percentage of babies come on their due date; a due date is just an estimation.
- Look at your due date as a five-week window of time rather than a specific date.
- Have a few answers ready for if people ask you about your due date – it takes pressure off and reduces the enquiries.
- Ask your midwife about your risks if you go overdue – are there other options for you?

Your postnatal plan

YOUR POSTNATAL TIME needs a bit of planning too. It is hard to think about this when you are pregnant because giving birth is naturally at the forefront of your mind. At the same time, it is important that you think and plan out a few things because there is even more to do when baby arrives. To have the best chance at having the birth you want, you need to plan for and have access to the right conditions – it is exactly the same for a smoother postnatal period. We need to create conditions to help you flourish as a new mother and having a plan is part of building strong foundations for your beautiful new family. Here are a few ideas about what to plan for postnatally.

PLAN TO REST

As a rule of thumb, you should avoid making any plans to do things for the first week after birth. Get back into bed whenever you feel you need to. During the second week make plans, but mainly with your sofa. I'm not joking when I say that. Stress can come from being somewhere and thinking you should be somewhere else. If you plan for at least two weeks at home and you feel like leaving your postnatal sanctuary then, that's fine. But, if you plan to meet a friend for lunch or have family round (see page 148) and don't have the energy to, then you may become stressed because you haven't met your own expectations or you feel obliged to leave your sanctuary. Rest is a crucial part of your recovery and you won't regret making the most of it.

MAKING A PLAN

Making a birth plan is a good idea, as we have seen, but have you thought about making a postnatal plan? You don't necessarily need to write out answers like a birth plan, unless you want to, but make sure you fully consider each point. Here is a list of questions and suggestions to help you:

Your support squad

Try to have a think about who's doing what and when. There may be things you already know for sure, like a date your partner is going back to work. Any set dates and information like this is useful because you can plan around it. You could start a 'people to call upon' list now. This sounds silly, but when you're sleep-deprived and have brain fog it can be hard to remember who to call and who will be available when. Having a clear list with names and numbers alone can help you feel supported and *feeling* supported is essential in those early days. You may never call the people on that list, but knowing you have those people at your fingertips can sometimes be good enough. Maternity helplines are listed in the resources on page 338.

Plan your home handover

Think about things that you may need relief from. There will be things that you normally do that no one else does, whether it is ordering the groceries online, paying bills or doing the nursery run. List the stuff you normally get on with but will need to hand over for a bit. Physical recovery goes hand in hand with mental recovery, so don't expect to do everything you could do before. Your autopilot might not be operating as well because you need to look after someone else now, and it is normal to forget the things you usually remember. Your mind needs rest too. Your mind and your body are so closely connected, even though modern-day life can encourage us to view our bodies as vehicles to get us places, to meetings or events, new motherhood means taking care of yourself entirely. Women often try to keep up with everything they normally do, then feel like a failure when they haven't done it. That's because it's *impossible* to do it all, especially just after giving birth, so rather than set yourself up to feel like you failed, plan for what you need help with.

Choose and use your visitors wisely

Who's coming, when and why? I tell all new mums to view visiting time as an opportunity for an extra pair of hands to help you get stuff done. You are your baby's main lifeline. Visiting is not a chance for them to sit on the sofa and cuddle your baby while you frantically shove stuff in the washing machine and make them tea. You certainly shouldn't be making visitors anything, other than a list of things to do.

You'll have a limited amount of time and energy to give in a day (and that's putting it mildly) so make sure you spend your precious energy wisely. Accepting visitors is allowing people into your postnatal sanctuary; only let those in who are willing to offer help. Prepare to set boundaries – the first few weeks are ever so precious. You and your baby aren't a source of entertainment for anyone else. You may need to discuss this with your partner ahead of time so that they can help and be the gatekeeper of your postnatal sanctuary. It's useful to discuss now rather than wonder why their cousin and her three kids can't come and see the baby yet. This may sound a bit harsh right now, but when the time comes you'll be thankful you planned like this.

'I cringe when I remember when my sister gave birth and I was at her house cuddling the baby thinking I was being helpful ... while waiting for her to make me dinner. I never made her a cup of tea. Or ran her a bath. Or told her it was going to be okay. I'd brought a teddy bear and thought I had done my bit. I had no idea how to honour myself after birth. It has taken FOUR babies for me to realise how absolutely vital it is to nuture a newborn mother for those first 40 days after birth. How SHE needs to be the focus. More so than the baby.'

Claire, mum of four, @jetsetmama

THE IMPORTANCE OF SUPPORT

'You'll hear so often that the birth of a baby is also the birth of a mother (and father!). We believe this is so true, and from our experiences as mothers and grandmother – we personally understand that enormous transition from "me" to "us". It matters, and whatever your individual circumstances, your background or position, having a baby is life-changing.

'The thing is, each mother or parent feels differently. There's no "normal" or expected reaction to giving birth. As experienced midwives we've been privileged to share the moments of the first union, at all types of births, the joy, the (sometimes) sadness, the shock, or the slow-to-get-going due to separation. Whatever the situation, we both fully support the notion that mothers and parents need love and support to help the process of attachment and "responsive parenting". So we encourage you to form your circle of support during pregnancy – enlist family and friends to come alongside you and be part of your journey. From a phone chat to a visit, from making a cup of tea to providing a meal, it really makes a difference.

'But remember the first few days are for you and your baby – try to make space to recover, to heal and to get to know each other. Your supporters can help by cooking for you, cleaning your home if you want it, or giving you whatever makes you feel good. You may want someone to take your baby for a walk, or cuddle her while you sleep, or you may absolutely not want any of these suggestions. This is your body and your baby, you call the shots Mama!'

Dr Sheena Byrom OBE and Dr Anna Coonan-Byrom, Senior Midwifery Lecturer, Midwife, Director All4Maternity

GET SOME PAID HELP

If you can afford to, put a little more money aside for a cleaner to come in for the first month after birth – once a week is great but it could be just twice in that first month if you need to keep costs down. Even if they just come that once or twice, it can really help take the pressure off everyone at home.

FEEDING PLAN FOR YOU

Eating properly with nourishing food in these first few weeks is so important for your wellbeing, and will help aid your healing and recovery. Salty and sugary snacks are fine for a quick fix but you don't want your postnatal diet to be reliant on them for fuel.

Try and set some time aside on maternity leave to cook and freeze some decent meals to enjoy and, of course, your partner can do this too. Again, let them know this ahead of time to avoid any 'hanger' disagreements. There are some suggested postnatal meals on page 139, and see page 268 for more on postnatal nutrition.

People are often happy to help cook if they know it will be welcome. If people ask what you might want as a gift, why not suggest a home-cooked meal?

FEEDING PLAN FOR BABY

How do you plan on feeding your baby? What support do you have to achieve your feeding goals? Who do you know who has fed a baby this way? Start thinking about your plan and once again, build in support early on. What does your partner think about your plan? They need to know as much as you do about feeding so that they can help and fully support your feeding plan. Regardless of how you feed, it is still a team effort, and it is very reassuring for mums when their partner is right by their side helping make up bottles or helping to make sure the latch is good and you are comfortable with pillows, water etc. On page 285 we will cover feeding fully.

'I'm a midwife from Devon and I moved away after meeting my now husband at university. My family (apart from my mum who died when I was 19) still live in Devon. Pregnancy-wise, everything was normal and low-risk and I had a water-birth; no complications, just a very long and painful back labour (baby was back-to-back until second stage). I spent a lot of time on the pregnancy and what labour and birth I would like, but I gave no thought to what going home with a baby would actually be like. I think I just presumed everything would be fine because I'm a midwife and see babies all the time! This was the first shock; I couldn't believe I was responsible for this tiny human.

'The feeding over those first weeks did not go to plan either. I had planned on breastfeeding, and antenatally I had expressed a lot of colostrum and she fed on me twice in hospital. I initially noticed a tongue tie, but didn't think much of it because we don't do anything at our Trust for at least seven days. However, over the next few days her latch became worse and she couldn't attach. I went back in to see the BF support but they couldn't get her to attach either, but referred me to the Lactation Consultant for tongue tie the following week, but by the end of the week we'd moved onto formula. The whole issue of feeding was just an emotional rollercoaster. Again, I assumed I'd just be able to do it but I wish I had planned this more.'

Ellie, midwife and first-time mum

PLAN FOR PROGRESS NOT PERFECTION

Spoiler alert: the perfect newborn and postpartum period don't exist. When new mums plan for 'progress' rather than 'perfection', they feel more positive, strong and capable at the end of the day, rather than chasing 'perfection'. For example, if you are having initial challenges with feeding your baby, look for the progress you're making. If your baby needs to go to special care, focusing on the daily progress gets you through tough times. No matter what your situation is, if you ditch the idea of perfection and just focus on your and your baby's unique progress, you are winning. That's why many athletes or runners mainly focus on their personal best (PB); they don't compare their PB to Mo Farah because they would constantly feel disappointed. The focus is on what they have personally achieved and how great their progress is. Beyoncé said in an interview: 'I'm competitive really with myself, honestly ... really my reference is, I go back to myself. I don't like to compete with anyone else.' You're on your own unique journey. Take one step at a time.

'A journey of a thousand miles begins with
a single step'

— LAO TZU

A LITTLE BOX OF CARE

This is a chance to buy yourself a few treats and essentials to enjoy in the first hazy days after baby arrives. Find a nice box or basket and add a few things that are just for you – a lot of women that do this then leave it under their bed. This could be some sweet treats, dark chocolate, a candle, some facial oil or a leave-in hair conditioner. After you have had a baby it can feel like a lot of your hair is falling out – don't worry this is normal and a lot of women get it. To help the condition of your hair you can try a leave-in conditioner or just some coconut oil and leave it tied up for a few hours to soak in. Popping a candle on (safely) and biting into some dark chocolate can make the night feeds that little bit more enjoyable too. You might also want to pop in some arnica if you would usually use that for pain and bruising and stock up on painkillers such as paracetamol and ibuprofen (as long as you aren't allergic) because you can get quite swollen and sore, especially if you have a wound.

MAKING TIME FOR EACH OTHER

Some of my patients and friends have done this and I thought it a nice one to share with you. Think about setting a checking-in alarm on your phone, about every five days, to check in with your partner. You may not need it or naturally do this anyway, but make sure you plan to check in with each other regularly and offer empathetic listening. Days can quickly become weeks when you are new parents, and good communication is ever so important (see page 326). You might not notice how all-consumed you are with your baby, but your partner will feel it most.

LET'S TALK ABOUT POO

Although this may seem like a weird one to consider now, you need to think about your first postnatal poo. Many women get quite (understandably) distressed about having their first poo after giving birth, especially if you have had stitches or a wound. If you get constipated, this can trap wind and it can be really uncomfortable. Midwives will ask you, 'Have you opened your bowels yet?' meaning, have you had a poo yet? Here are the key things you need to do now to help you have your first successful number two.

- Pre-labour stay active, practise yoga (see page 115) and go for a walk at least three times a week as it helps with circulation and digestion.
- Drink hot water and lemon first thing in the morning to kick-start your digestive system. Sip water regularly throughout the day to stay well hydrated.
- You need roughage to assist with digestion. Eat fruits and vegetables and wholegrain products like spelt, brown rice and oats. Sprinkle your salads, smoothies and breakfast cereals with added extras such as crushed linseeds, chia seeds and prunes.
- If you're on it, take iron with orange juice; it helps with absorption and reduces constipation.
- Keep a small footstool in the bathroom. Placing your feet on the stool while on the toilet reduces the need to push or strain, which most women are nervous to do, so why not buy this now and give it a try?
- Use your down-breathing (see page 185); this can help you avoid straining and to relax more on the loo.

KEY POINTS

- Prepare your personal postnatal sanctuary and stay at home as much as you want to.
- Set boundaries on the amount of visitors. Your partner can help manage the flow of visitors.
- Plan some meals ahead of time and, if offered, accept food from visitors.
- The housework can wait – rest whenever you get the chance to. If you can, pay for a cleaner to help, even for a short time.
- Plan to treat yourself well with a care box, and let yourself recover during this time.

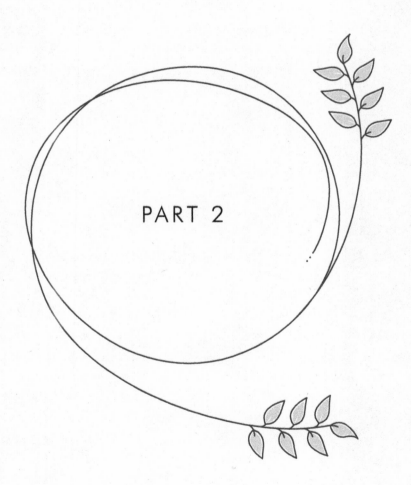

PART 2

Your Positive Birth

Welcome to the birth section! Here we will cover the key things you need to know and understand about birth. I have kept it as concise as possible and will share with you only the things most women need to know. For any more in-depth questions about your individual circumstances, make sure to talk to your midwife or doctor.

I won't get started again on the portrayal of birth in the media, but to be honest, it's mostly a load of nonsense. My family can't bear to watch any birth scenes with me as I annoyingly ruin the film by going off on a rant. Unfortunately, most women I meet have only seen the media's version of what birth looks like.

The truth about birth is that some elements are unpredictable, and there is no 'one rule fits all'. But if you take anything from the entire birth section, take this. **Nobody fails at labour and birth.** I didn't want to, it wasn't an option for me or it was best to, are the best phrases when referring to any change of plan.

The experience of being a midwife has allowed me to meet women from so many different walks of life, most ethnic origins and various cultures. This has taught me that there are a *lot* of ways to have a positive birth experience, and no one thing works for everyone. That said, I have noticed that the women who have positive births seem to share some common traits, regardless of age, ethnicity, birth setting or type. These are a combination of five things:

1. Understanding the birthing body and support of natural female physiology – regardless of birth type.
2. Use of mind-management tools such as breathing and relaxation techniques – regardless of birth type.
3. Mum in control, with trusted birth experts encouraging, supporting and guiding, if necessary.
4. Looking at the *individual* circumstances before, and in combination with, treatment, if needed.
5. Prevention of complications, such as dehydration, positioning and stalled labour.

Having a more positive birth is about creating an experience in which you are fully informed and understand your options. You need to understand how your body works during birth so that you can work with it. Here we will run through the most common situations, and aim to crush any fears – your worst enemy in labour. Some mums have very kindly shared their birth stories for us throughout this section to read too.

Your toolkit

WHERE THE MIND goes the body tends to follow. This section is about 'tools' that can help you manage labour, work with your body, release fear and create the best mindset to deal with any situation in the most positive way possible. This section is all about you creating a toolkit to use during pregnancy and labour, and this starts with a positive mindset, so let's start with the most positive fact about labour:

The majority of the time spent in labour is **resting** – the time spent relaxing and doing nothing is about 70 per cent. This is because most women in established labour will have around three contractions in 10 minutes, each lasting up to one minute. So, in a 10-minute period about seven of those minutes are spent resting. As reassuring as that is to know, I also appreciate there is a lot more that goes on inside your head before and during labour. Fear is a big issue during the lead up to birth, so let's talk about this now.

SAYING GOODBYE TO FEAR

Women often become hyper-aware of their safety during pregnancy and birth, which is entirely natural. Things you weren't worried about before now play on repeat in your mind. If you can learn to overcome fear, or develop tools to manage it, with renewed confidence a whole new world opens up and your entire perception changes. All fears about birth hold you back, but they don't have to any more. Fear and anticipation of an experience are often worse than the experience itself. When you focus on a bad outcome, you feel like you're living in it in those moments, and so does your body. Fear during birth can make everything tougher.

'The only thing we have to fear is fear itself'

— FRANKLIN D ROOSEVELT

Your mind believes what you tell it. Next time you're hungry, picture your favourite food vividly. You won't even need to see or smell it but your mouth waters. Pizza gets me every time — even when I'm not particularly hungry! As the mind and body are so well connected, I've suggested to some of my patients that they try the 'brain dump' and unpack their own thoughts.

If you're scared about something, start with what is going on in your mind right now. Write down any of your fears in a notebook. By doing this, those fears are no longer in an internal neurological circuit – firing off around your brain. That old saying, 'a problem shared is a problem halved' is so true, but you don't need to share your fears with someone if you don't want to; writing it down or admitting this to yourself is a good place to start.

Once you have identified your fears, interrogate them, and find out just how they got there. In order to change something, we first need to understand it, so ask yourself: Is this a deep-rooted fear you've held for many years or is this a more recently learned fear? Is it rational or have you jumped to a conclusion?

Take a moment to really think about why you fear something. If you have any specific fears or worries that have developed about or during your pregnancy, simply talking to your midwife or doctor can help. Stuff can come up that you have been suppressing and just chatting through it can dissolve your worry. I find that a lot of fear surrounding birth comes from horrible stories other people have told my patients, or what the media tells us about birth.

Take any of those stories that have scared you straight to the dumping ground. If you wrote it down, physically screw it up and chuck it out. The experience you heard about, or read about, is not yours, and it will never be, because no two births are the same.

Fear that comes from a previous loss or traumatic event is slightly different as this is your personal experience. If you have lost a baby remember that this is a *different pregnancy at a different time*. Until you have your baby in your arms an element of fear may still be there, but being open about your fear and previous experience and addressing it can reduce the power fear may have over you, your experience of having *this* baby at this *time*. Always talk to your midwife about how you are feeling to help release fear and address if you need any further support during your pregnancy. See page 233 for Hannah's experience of her pregnancy and birth with her rainbow baby.

You are going to understand all of your options, you are going to be in control, and you are going to be well supported.

'Every living being will experience fear, it's inevitable and unavoidable. But you can go beyond the menace of fear. It's possible to use fear to transcend your imagined limitations and find your true Self.'

— MOOJI

After you have addressed, dissolved or dumped your fear you don't want anyone else to dump their bad experience back into your brain. Any time anyone starts offloading, tell them you don't want to talk about it right now. Instead, maybe let them know you're happy to talk about it after you've had your baby. There is a time and place for debriefing, and that is not with you during your pregnancy – thank you very much! As Ina May Gaskin says: 'It is bad manners to be scaring pregnant women', so don't feel bad about shutting them down because your psychological wellbeing is more important than *their* desire to tell you about *their* experience.

Women and their families worry about all kinds of things, but the top two most common fears I hear are not having a healthy baby and pain in labour. Let's pull these top two apart right now, and then move on to creating your positive toolkit.

AN EXTRA NOTE ON FEAR

If you are developing, or have known, tokophobia (a significant fear of childbirth), this brain-dumping may not help you. Talk to your midwife about your other options as soon as possible.

THE IDEA OF A 'HEALTHY' BABY

In the Western world, we are extremely lucky to have access to amazing maternity healthcare, treatment and life-saving technology. We are always working to prevent ill-health, rather than wait to cure. Midwives, doctors and other healthcare professionals work tirelessly to improve healthcare and long-term outcomes.

Being fearful that something may happen to your baby is *natural* but it's not *helpful,* because fear and trust cannot co-exist. Your baby is in the safest and best place for you both; a trained professional will be caring for you and someone you trust will be with you. What is worrying going to do to help you have a healthy baby? It might give you a distorted, negative view of your own ability, use up precious brainpower and energy mulling over 'what-ifs', which you really don't need! If you have a concern, worry or gut feeling something isn't right, always call your midwife. But, unless that is the case, try to let go of this fear and stay rooted in reality so you can build trust in your own ability and your midwife.

There is an interesting (and real tear-jerker) TED Talk by Karni Liddell, who is a Paralympic swimmer from Australia. She makes us deeply question the desire for a 'healthy baby'. She asks if having a certain body automatically equates to being happy and successful, does it guarantee you joy and prosperity or even health? This statement really made me question my own perception of what we perceive to be 'healthy':

'There are plenty of 'able-bodied' people that are miserable, not healthy, overly happy or successful. So why is it okay to assume disability is lesser than, and associate disability as being an automatic reduction in the status as a person? Why is it okay to say that a disability is your worst nightmare? I think the most disabling thing we do to ourselves is this quest for "normality" and hunger for perfection.'

She concludes her point by reminding us that, to a certain extent, we can't always control 'being healthy' so why don't we chuck that word aside and replace it with wanting a happy baby.

THINKING ABOUT PAIN?

You have options available to help with any pain you may experience. There is so much that you can do to manage your own pain, and we are going to cover the best, most researched, and proven pain-management tools soon. But always remember that, if needed, you can use medication and move on to an epidural; it is perfectly okay to do that if you want to. Labour will be manageable with your unique tool box, all the pain-relief medication you have access to, and the support you have available from midwives and your birth partner. **You can do this.**

Reframing – how you think about a challenge – is used by celebrities, top CEOs and professional athletes. Runners use the reframing technique all the time. They tell themselves how much they love hills and reframe how they look at running uphill. Guess what? Those that use reframing experience the run differently, and have a better chance of running to the top of that hill!

When it comes to the pain of labour, reframing how you think about it can really change your experience of it. Here are some suggestions for you to think about:

- Contractions are useful and are working towards a life-changing moment as they come and go.
- Contractions are different to any other type of pain the human body experiences. If you break your leg it hurts because you aren't meant to

move a broken leg – your body is protecting you from further injury. The 'pain' of contractions is positive, because you *need* them to have your baby. There is an end goal in sight and each contraction is getting you closer to meeting your baby.

- There is a difference between natural and unnatural pain. It is an unfair comparison when people say things like, 'Well you wouldn't have a tooth out without painkillers.' No, Sherlock, you wouldn't want to do this. But the pain of having a tooth extracted is an unnatural pain – even if it's necessary – something has gone wrong in order for you to need it out. That is different to a normal, healthy and natural birth.

I'm not saying birth and labour is in any way pain-free, but it is a different *kind* of pain, possibly the most useful pain you'll ever experience. It's useful to note too, that not all women experience pain in labour. I have looked after women who have used reframing who have said: 'It was powerful and hard work but it wasn't *painful*. I would do it all again.'

A WAVE VISUALISATION

Let's try a bit of reframing and a useful visualisation now.

Imagine it is a beautiful day and you are at the beach. You are lying on a lilo a little away from the shore. You can see the beach and your favourite people are on the shore. In order to get to them, all you need to do is to relax and let the lilo carry you there on the waves. The tide carries you, each wave is bringing you closer and closer to the shore. During the pauses between waves, you are totally relaxed and at peace, enjoying the calm, peaceful ocean before the next wave comes to carry you closer ...

Birth is a little bit like the waves on the beach. To meet your baby, you need to relax and go with the waves (contractions). They carry you there more easily if you allow them to. Each wave is bringing you that little bit closer to your baby.

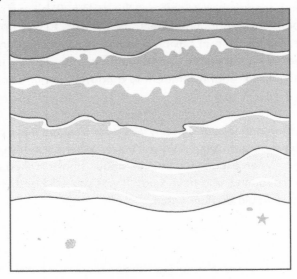

CREATING A HOME IN HOSPITAL

If hospital environments scare you, but it is safer for you to give birth there, then you can use 'reframing'. Try to think about how lucky you are to be able to give birth in such a safe place for you and your baby. Focus more on the ways that you can still create the birth you want, and think about all the things that will make your transition from home to hospital less daunting. This could be something like bringing your own pillow and blanket in, a picture to pop on the bedside table, or one in your bag to look at when you want to. These little things really help you to feel more positive and at ease.

The significance of smell
Our sense of smell is so underrated yet it is intrinsic to almost everything we experience. For example, without our sense of smell, taste is only salty, sour,

sweet and bitter. We are heavily dependent on smells to taste flavour. Smell seriously improves our quality of life. This is all down to what is called the olfactory bulb, which begins in the nose and runs to the bottom of the brain. The two areas it is connected to are the amygdala and hippocampus and are thought to be mostly involved in processing memories and emotion. The interesting part is that our other senses (visual, sound and touch) don't pass through these sections of the brain, which may explain why we have such strong reactions to familiar scents. Ever sprayed an old perfume and been taken straight back to that time in your life? Weird, isn't it. Someone sprayed 'Charlie Red' in a shop aisle recently, and I was instantly transported back to being 15 years old in the PE changing rooms!

During labour we should be using this strong memory link to our advantage and create new memories attached to smells. My suggestion is take a scented bath towards the end of pregnancy – only use oils that are safe for your gestation. Run a nice warm bath (or tepid if it's summer and you're sticky), pop a drop of lavender oil in, and as you swish the water around, take some nice, deep breaths and enjoy the feeling of calm, private, peace. If you do this regularly you will start to associate the smell of lavender with calmness and safety. Have the lavender oil with you during labour and you can tap into this feeling through the scent.

Aromatherapy use in labour (especially if you are in a hospital environment) can be a real game changer, and can help to reduce anxiety, nervousness and even nausea. The NHS have started investing in training midwives in aromatherapy because of its beneficial impact on labour and birth.

Here are the most popular essential oils and their properties:

Clary sage – one of the most popularly used oils in labour, it helps with muscle spasms and is thought to aid dilation of the cervix.

Chamomile – is a lovely soothing oil that aids relaxation.

Sweet citrus – uplifting, it can help with depression and calms nerves, and most other oils blend well with citrus too.

Lavender – one of my general favourites, it is an antiseptic and is known to have a lovely calming effect too. I mix it with peppermint and grapeseed oil and use this as a massage oil.

Frankincense – one of my personal favourites, it is most commonly used during 'transition', the time when you are almost ready to push. It is calming, soothing and a meditative oil.

Jasmine – known for its antiseptic, uterotonic and restorative properties, this oil is quite strong and should not be used before 37 weeks.

Note: Essential oils are powerful so do discuss using them with a midwife or an aromatherapist. Do a patch test before using on your skin.

Dim the lights

One of the most exciting and recent advances in the relationship between modern medicine and ancient wisdom is a trial using melatonin to induce women. Melatonin is the hormone that helps to regulate our sleep–wake cycle and induce sleep. It is produced naturally and released by the pineal gland. Melatonin responds to light and dark and is known as the 'Dracula of hormones', because it's released in darkness and is scared off by light.

A recent trial in Australia confirms what many of us thought: low lighting helps labour progression.

Melatonin encourages the production of oxytocin, which is essential for labour and we will cover other oxytocin enhancers on page 176. Research shows that the myometrial tissue (muscle tissue in the uterus) becomes responsive to melatonin's prompts during labour. Using biopsy samples, scientists found the tissue expressed the melatonin 2 (MT2) receptor during labour, something that was not found in a non-pregnant uterus. What this tells us is that when the lighting is low or dim in the birthing room, your body has the opportunity to progress labour normally using its natural workings that it has especially prepared during your pregnancy. How clever is that!

I have also noticed that dim lighting usually means quieter voices. I guess because we associate darkness with sleeping, and we don't want to wake the person up. This is perfect in labour because when you are in the zone you don't want to be 'woken up' or startled out of it unnecessarily. Dim lighting also helps women feel less observed, especially if they are hardly wearing anything or are completely naked (both very common). You can request dim lighting in all hospital birth settings and ask for us to work around you. There have been plenty of times when I have dimmed the lights at 'high-risk' births and had a lamp only directing light on the monitors or paperwork I need to see. The entire room doesn't have to be bright clinical lights, unless there is a true emergency or you are in theatre.

MASSAGE AND TOUCH

Massage and touch can both help to ease contractions and can generally make you feel more relaxed (if you like it, of course!). Massage is known to increase blood supply, decrease heart rate, help with lymphatic drainage, increase oxytocin and decrease stress hormones like cortisol.

You don't need a professional masseuse in the birthing room with you; you can get your birth partner to do it. And they'll love knowing that they are helping in some way. Massage is usually a case of exploration and experiment but most women prefer a firm lower back massage rather than a light shoulder rub. Grapeseed oil is the recommended massage oil for labour – you can also add essential oils of your choice to the oil for maximum affect.

BACK
MASSAGE
MOTION

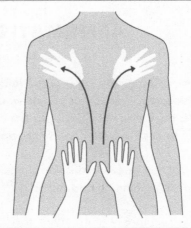

1. Starting at the base of your lower back, with a hand either side of the spine, use your hands to massage up and out. Imagine the spine is a tree trunk and their fingers are the palm tree leaves, spreading outwards.
2. Repeat as often as you like!

WARM FLANNELS

Compresses placed on the sacrum (the area just above your coccyx) during labour can provide some relief from contractions. You could add some aromatherapy oil too if you like (see page 167).

Women with an OP (occiput posterior or back-to-back) baby find this massage particularly comforting, but it can take its toll on the birth partner's hands! A hand-held massager can come in handy here to give their hands a break too.

Sometimes women who usually love a massage don't fancy one in labour, so touch, stroking and hand-holding are great replacements. A study by pain researcher Dr Goldstein revealed that when an empathetic partner holds the hand of a woman in pain, their heart and respiratory rates sync and her pain is reduced. This could be a partner or a midwife. Dr Goldstein led this study after his hand-holding really seemed to help his wife, and thought that touch could be a tool for communicating empathy, resulting in an analgesic, or pain-killing, effect.

AFFIRMATIONS

Not so long ago affirmations (positive self-talk) weren't very popular or taught in antenatal education. Sometimes people would laugh or brush off the power of affirmations. My friend once said, 'It's not about wishful thinking ... I need some real help to deal with what's coming, damn it!'

The greatest athletes to ever walk the planet and many global A-listers use affirmations, positive thinking and self-talk.

Muhammad Ali would say affirmations like, 'I am the greatest' because he was a talented boxer willing to dedicate hours to training – he knew he could be the greatest. It was a realistic affirmation for him and then he put the work in. Affirmations have helped many people reach a goal, get to the top of their game and dig deep in times of self-doubt.

Although affirmations are now making their way into birth, it is worth squashing some common misconceptions about them – they aren't just for hippies or wishful thinkers. But on the flip side, simply believing you can doesn't guarantee you can. Some aspects of birth are unpredictable and all the affirmations in the world can't change that. The sweet spot is focusing on realistic and honest positive self-talk that is unique to you. Affirmations work best when:

1. They are realistic for you.
2. You believe them.
3. You learn what to do.

I have listed some suggested affirmations for you but it is worth creating your own that are meaningful and feel right for you, because you need these to believe these with sincerity. Then make your chosen affirmations into posters, pop them around your room, next to or on the bathroom mirror, and say them out loud or go over them as often as possible. You may also want to bring affirmations with you wherever you give birth – especially if you need to travel in the car. Sometimes the car journey in can be a little daunting or uncomfortable as you have to stay still. Having your affirmations handy can help you stay in a positive mindset:

I will make the best decision for me and my baby

I trust my true instincts and listen to my body

I breathe in confidence and trust, I breathe out fear and tension

I trust my body

My baby is the best birthing partner

I am safe and feel calm within

I am powerful

Women worldwide are birthing with me

I am open

POSITIVE SOCIAL MEDIA

Consider putting positive social-media accounts such as @thepositivebirth movement @birthwithoutfear, @melissajeanbabies @hannahbphotographyuk @empoweredbirthproject, podcasts, birth stories and birth photography in your labour toolkit too. Open up to social media that is going to support you and build upon your positive mindset. This opening up creates a new narrative about birth and gives you the opportunity to see birth in a positive way. Ina May Gaskin has a great TED Talk on her experiences as a midwife 'reducing fear of birth in US culture' and there's a golden oldie video on YouTube that I recommend you watch called 'Birth in the squatting position', with many different women giving birth naturally. Most women having a baby have not actually *seen* a birth, and on many social media accounts and YouTube you can watch beautiful births. You may then find that you are more able to come up with visualisations when you have seen births that inspire you.

KEY POINTS

- Seventy per cent of labour is resting.
- Face your fears – identify what's bothering you and why. And then you can work out what to do with them.
- Where the mind goes the body tends to follow – put together your unique positive mental labour toolkit.
- Seek out positive social media to build your own narrative of what labour and birth is like.

Step out of the way and trust your body

UNDERSTANDING HOW BIRTH works and working with your natural female physiology may help you to get closer to the birth you have in mind. It is surprising how little most of us know or are taught about birth, other than the ingrained message of 'it's going to hurt'. As we've taken that fear to the dumping ground (see page 160), it is time to fill the space you have created with knowledge and confidence. The birthing female body is incredibly powerful and it is about time every woman knew how it really works, regardless of where or how you have your baby. So, this section will explain how to help your labouring body, no matter where you give birth.

THE SCIENCE BEHIND THE BIRTHING BRAIN

The human brain plays an important role in protecting us, processing new information and helping us overcome obstacles. The capabilities of the brain are extraordinary. Neuroscientists have shown that our brains are 'soft-wired' and are capable of neuroplasticity; this means that we can 'rewire' our brains. There have been cases where people who have suffered serious brain injuries have returned to their normal self with the right support and rehabilitation. My all-time favourite TED Talk by Jill Bolte Taylor, 'My Stroke of Insight', shows us just how able and adaptable our beautiful brains are.

A healthy brain is always capable of learning. This allows us to change, grow and to overcome our fears. I could waffle on about this but let's get to the point about birth. Understanding the basics of how your brain works during labour can really help prevent a stalled or slower labour; speeding up labour is not guaranteed, but understanding the brain definitely helps.

There are three main sections in the brain: the neocortex or 'human brain', the mammalian brain and the reptile brain. The neocortex and the mammalian brain are the two main parts of the brain that impact every woman's birth (the reptile or cerebellum part of your brain controls the basic body functions and primitive survival circuits).

Your brain in action

The neocortex is the most modern part of the brain, the managing director, and it is useful for daily tasks like planning for things, reasoning and conscious thought. It controls what sets us apart from other species. However, in some situations we need to slow it down and stop it from taking over so another part of our brain (mammalian) can function at its best. The perfect example of a time when you need to 'turn down' your neocortex is during sex. What were you thinking about when you had the best sex of your life? Were you worrying about who could hear you or if something went wrong? Probably not; you were most likely absorbed in the moment and *not thinking*. You can't enjoy sex properly if your mind starts wandering or worrying because your neocortex has now become active and your mammalian brain can't take over and relax.

This is the same concept with labour and birth. Labour and birth are primal and instinctive. You can help encourage it all along with the right company and environment but it's not something you actively do; labour and birth are something that happens.

There's a really simple secret to an easier labour: **when your mind stays relaxed your body gets on with what it needs to do, allowing hormonal synchronicity.**

When relaxed, your brain has the best opportunity to send all of the right signals to help your body labour and does all the work for you. Just like an orgasm – you can't force it. Birth (like orgasm) will usually only happen in the right environment, when the mind lets go and you're completely relaxed. In terms of how the brain is working, you're turning off your 'thinking' – or the neocortical activity – giving your physical reflexes a chance to work. In the context of birth, this is known as the 'fetal ejection reflex'. This is when a baby is born with no conscious effort or voluntary movements and it explains why women can give birth even whilst in a coma. The good news is that it doesn't just happen when women are unconscious; I have seen this happen many times with women who have really been able to mentally step out of the way, go within, and trust their body.

When the mind is stimulated, over-active or fearful, the body slows down labour. Our conscious mind literally gets in the way. This response is an evolutionary defence mechanism and can happen even when there is only a *perceived* threat. Imagine a labouring woman thousands of years ago, vulnerable to dangerous prey: if she needed to escape, her body would need to stop labouring. The body reacts to the information you are giving it. For example, you see a tiger, the stress hormones are activated, oxytocin is reduced, labour stops/slows and the woman has the chance to get away. Ever had a nightmare and woken up really believing what happened and feeling full of fear, with your heart racing and sweating? It takes a while to calm down, doesn't it? That perceived threat is an example of how powerful the mind and imagination are, and the effects they have on the physical body. The body doesn't yet have the ability to tell the difference between a perceived threat and a real threat so it treats them the same.

You **think** there is a threat: stress response activated
You **see** a real threat: stress response activated

Sometimes women don't allow themselves to let go during labour and birth. They worry about making noises, swearing, farting and pooing. Let anything out that wants to come out. Honestly, midwives couldn't give a damn, and there's not a lot that I haven't heard, smelt or seen, so if you're worrying about what we'll think, please don't.

Diverting energy to your human brain by analysing or worrying doesn't only slow labour down, but it also wastes your precious mental energy. Have you ever spent an hour sitting down with someone who needs to offload and felt completely drained afterwards? That's because they have been sucking up your mental energy and taking your focus to various toxic or emotionally draining topics. This kind of mental exhaustion is exactly the kind you want to avoid during labour.

Your mammalian brain is partly responsible for sending signals to your body that affect the natural progression of labour. These trigger a release of the birth-dependent hormones, oxytocin, beta-endorphins – your natural pain relievers – and melatonin. In conjunction with some other things (like your baby's position – remember your UFO position), oxytocin leads labour progression. Oxytocin is released by your nervous system so it isn't something you can consciously control but you can encourage it in many ways (see below). Even though oxytocin has so much power it is still a very shy leader and will only come out and work its magic when you turn your neocortex down and provide the right environment. Another way I explain this to my patients is to imagine the type of environment you prefer to have sex in. Perhaps dim lighting, maybe some candles, a bit of background music and in private. Now imagine having sex in bright lights, with people watching, clinical smells, random voices and noises right outside the door. You wouldn't be able to relax, would you?

THE BIRTH HORMONE

We have around 100 hormones in our bodies and as far as we know the main hormone responsible for labour is oxytocin, aka the 'love hormone'. You probably would have felt that fuzzy rush of oxytocin during sex, while having a snuggle on the sofa or even when you've had your hair played with. Anything that makes you feel safe and relaxed can release oxytocin. Once I was lost and having a crap day. I asked someone for directions in the street and this sweet older lady spoke really calmly, with a gentle smile, finishing with 'Are you going to be okay getting there, my love?' I felt all fuzzy and warm – but then thought to myself: did I just get a rush of oxytocin from directions?!

There are many ways to encourage oxytocin during labour and birth:

- **Relax**
  Your body needs to be relaxed. Tension increases pain, which increases fear and therefore stress hormones, preventing the natural flow of oxytocin.

Remember to keep your jaw nice and relaxed too. Massage helps many of us relax and some women like to try nipple stimulation to help them relax and release oxytocin. Give it a go if you like it!

- **Get comfortable**
  You need to get into positions where you feel most comfortable. Towards the end of labour this can be a challenge but as your labour progresses use your ball, go on your side, stand or lean over the bed and consider getting into water to help ease any backache. So many women get great relief from the pool. In early labour the bath can be nice but in established labour, or close to pushing, the pool is best as it allows you to get into positions you might not be able to on dry land and there's more room. It's not just about physically feeling comfortable, but mentally comfortable and confident too; remember that everything is flexible and you always have options. You don't 'have to' do anything.

- **Trust**
  You need to really trust your midwife, birth partners, your body and your baby to all work together as a team. This helps you to relax, feel comfortable and confident. See page 213 for more on how your baby is your best birth partner. Trust that you have and are doing everything you can to have a positive birth experience, and so is your body.

- **Be uninterrupted**
  Your mammalian brain should be uninterrupted by your neocortex, and being in a relaxed environment, without perceived 'threats', allows this.

The best birth environment for oxytocin to be released would have these features:

- **Dimly lit**
  As you know, melatonin affects labour progressing, and you have gained some extra receptors in pregnancy, so make the most use of them by keeping the room as dimly lit as possible. You can get flameless candles so you might want to bring those in with you if you're in an MLU or hospital.

- **Quiet**

  Loud noises or voices can be distracting and start off unnecessary communication with your neocortex, inhibiting that precious flow of oxytocin. Gentle music or hypnobirthing tracks can help prevent any internal noise. Quiet is also an environment most of us work best in, regardless of what we are doing.

- **Calm**

  A calm atmosphere reflects safety: wherever you are, you will have chosen the safest place for you and your baby. Make sure your birth partners keep the environment calm and keep themselves nice and calm. A person's demeanour can change the calmness of the environment.

- **Private**

  As oxytocin is shy it needs some privacy to perform at its best; even if you are in a hospital environment you can request as much privacy as possible. Keep your birth space private and intimate. If you are at home go to the room or place where you feel most sheltered, it is common for women having a home birth to plan to give birth in the lounge but end up on the bathroom floor. It shows how instinctive it is to seek privacy.

We have synthetic versions of oxytocin in hospital and we mainly rely on these versions to progress induction or speed up labour. We give you the synthetic version of oxytocin into your vein via an intravenous infusion (drip). One difference to understand is that when natural oxytocin is released in the body, it peaks and then drops back to a baseline. This is different from when we administer synthetic oxytocin, which is continuous. Your natural oxytocin is released into the brain, which is really beneficial to the birthing body and for the postnatal period. Synthetic oxytocin does not reach the brain. Some would argue that it doesn't matter if you have synthetic oxytocin or natural oxytocin because it's the same thing; we now know that *how* women get oxytocin does affect how it works in the body. That's not to say if you need the synthetic version for induction that it is bad. If your plan needs to change, the best thing you can do is accept your current circumstances and know that you are making the right decision for you and your baby at the time. If you have 'Synto', as us midwives call it, that doesn't mean everything else has to go out the window; in fact, your birth plan (see page 92) may be useful now, more than ever.

THE FEAR AND PAIN CYCLE AND HOW TO BREAK IT

Life is all about cycles: young to old, day to night, summer to winter. In birth, feeling fearful can bring you into an unhelpful cycle:

MUSCLE TENSION CAUSED BY FEAR RESULTS IN MORE PAIN, ULTIMATELY SLOWING PROGRESSION IN LABOUR

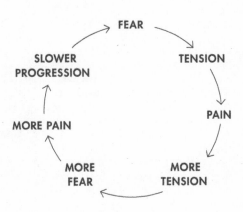

This cycle has been understood and documented as early as the 1900s. Dr Grantly Dick-Read is quoted as saying: 'Anything that disturbs the confidence and peacefulness of the mother disrupts the neuromuscular harmony of her labour ... In childbirth, fear and the anticipation of pain give rise to natural protective tensions in the body. Unfortunately, the natural muscular tension produced by fear also influences the muscles that close the womb and thus delay the progress of the labour and create pain ... The vicious circle of the fear – tension pain syndrome is responsible for the pain of labour.'

I disagree that fear is entirely responsible but there's no doubt in my mind that fear plays a significant role in pain perception.

Try to opt out of this cycle and instead opt into this more positive, 'forward' cycle:

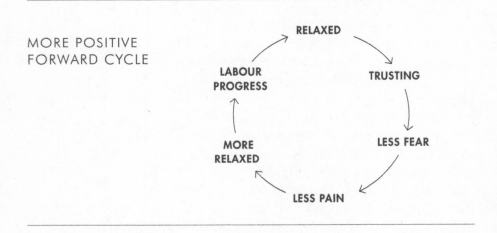

MORE POSITIVE
FORWARD CYCLE

RELAXED

TRUSTING

LESS FEAR

LESS PAIN

MORE RELAXED

LABOUR PROGRESS

Opting into the forward cycle is the best thing you can do if you want a calmer, shorter, more positive birth.

'So, how the hell do you "relax" when you're about to give birth to another human?' was what one of my heavily pregnant friends asked me after I started to explain birth biology and these cycles. I get it: it is totally unrealistic to know how to suddenly switch off the neocortex and 'just relax'. Your positive mental labour toolkit (see page 160) and oxytocin enhancers will help you massively but here are some other techniques to practise throughout your pregnancy.

THE LANGUAGE OF CONTRACTIONS

Recently, people have started to use the word 'surge' in place of 'contractions'. I understand that 'surge' may be a better word and has more positive connotations than ' contraction' but the word is deeply imbedded in maternity. It takes a long time to create change around language use, especially when clinical guidelines refer to the word contraction. It is likely that you will be asked about your contractions by professionals. Some mums are not familiar with the word surge either. To ensure that everyone understands what we are talking about, I will use the word contraction rather than surge in this book.

HOW TO SWITCH OFF YOUR ADVANCED BRAIN DURING BIRTH

Switching off the advanced part of the brain (the neocortex) during birth isn't necessarily easy but it is very doable with practice, more practice and you guessed it ... a bit more practice. I've seen many different women from different backgrounds at different kinds of births achieve a state of 'surrendered relaxation'.

Like anything worth achieving, the preparation usually takes longer than the event itself. An Olympic sprinter will spend years training, but their biggest achievement is over in seconds. People spend months, even years, planning a wedding and it's over in a day. The preparation for the event is what makes it. Whilst it is a great thing, positive thinking alone won't get you in the right state of mind. Of course, it's far better than negative thinking, but practising relaxation, breathing techniques and mindfulness regularly over time is what works.

You need to practise breathing and relaxation techniques daily. It's never too early or too late to start. There are different breathing and relaxation techniques out there but I'm a fan of hypnobirthing and am a qualified KG hypnobirthing teacher myself. I decided to do the formal training because the most peaceful births I have attended have been with women who have used hypnobirthing and the best thing about it is that it can be used for *any* birth.

HYPNOBIRTHING

Hypnobirthing is a form of evidence-based antenatal preparation that follows a logical and simple approach to mind management during birth. It uses breathing techniques, relaxation, touch, music, visualisations, self-hypnosis and education to help women have calmer, more positive births.

Although hypnobirthing has become popular in recent years, it has been around for a very long time – breathing, relaxation and self-hypnosis are ancient techniques that are used globally. Some NHS hospitals also offer hypnobirthing classes, there are various physical classes, digital packs, books and free YouTube videos to teach you about hypnobirthing. To some extent I think hypnobirthing is built into midwifery heritage because it is about working with your natural female physiology, and understanding the birthing brain and body.

BREATHING AFFECTS YOUR BRAIN

Breathing techniques slow down the autonomic nervous system, turning down stress hormones so they can't inhibit your flow of oxytocin. Relaxed breathing alone reduces fear and increases feelings of trust, because it slows down cerebral activity (the neocortex) and puts you in touch with your intuition; taking you from the physical to the internal. To the body, feelings are chemical messengers in the blood, so if we can influence your feelings we can change the chemicals in your blood. It is that simple and it can start with breathing.

Some women like to practise breathing techniques with their birth partners during labour because they feel as though someone is in the same mental space and is 'coaching' them through. Other women prefer to get into their own zone and use their own breathing and visualisation techniques. If you prefer to do this, breathe deeply and calmly, avoid panting like you see on TV. After practising a few times you'll get to know what works best for you. Whatever you choose, your aim is to help your body become as relaxed as possible and your mind to be as calm and peaceful as possible.

Your body spends the majority of labour softening, thinning and opening your cervix. The uterine muscle fibres are also drawing up and bunching at the top of your tummy. That's why midwives will always touch the top of your tummy to feel for your contractions even though you feel the sensation low down – we can only feel from the top. Calm breathing during labour helps this process to happen.

BREATHING IN LABOUR

Breathing can be a real help during birth; I recommend 'up-breathing' and 'down-breathing'. Up-breathing is what you'll be using from first contractions until you are ready to push, which is when you will switch to down-breathing (see page 185). Try to practise up-breathing every day between now and when baby arrives.

1. Sit comfortably, breathe in through your nose slowly and deeply.
2. Now breathe out through your mouth slowly through slightly parted lips; your out-breath needs to be a little longer than your in-breath.
3. Try this again, this time you can count, try in for 4 ... and out for 6, calmly, peacefully and softly.
4. Now try breathing in for 4 ... and breathing out for 8.
5. Choose whatever you are most comfortable with – out for 6 or 8 – and repeat this five times.
6. Notice how you now feel after just a short practise of this technique.

Five repetitions of up-breathing usually takes around one minute, which is about the same amount of time a contraction takes to build and peak and lower again. If you practise this daily, you will become familiar with these reps. When you're in labour you just need to get through five breaths for each contraction. **You can do it.**

When women are in this relaxed state of calm breathing or the 'zone', as many refer to it as, they experience less fear and pain, so their bodies labour more easily because they are being provided with oxytocin encouragers. Your contractions are far more effective when you're in this state too. I have seen first-time mums labour like they have had babies before while using these techniques. Some have gone from 2cm to fully dilated in just a few hours.

VISUALISATION IN LABOUR

Alongside breathing, visualisation can be very powerful during labour because the mind and body are able to work even more closely together – and that is the aim of the game. Imagine anything that helps you to focus on *up* and *out*, particularly on the longer out breath. Your cervix and muscles of the uterus need to open up. This is where you should really let go and release. Here is an example to try:

- Imagine the sunrise coming up and out from the sea on the horizon as you breathe in. Really picture the beautiful change in colours, then as the sun rises up into the sky breathe out. Stay focused on the peaceful movement of the sun and the tranquil, soft colours.
- Imagine a beautiful big oak tree sucking water up and breathing out. Imagine all the clean, renewing nutrients delicately reaching all the branches and leaves, calmly and peacefully moving up and out. Visualise this image as you breathe in and out.
- You could also use the lilo one we practised earlier if you liked it (see page 165).

I often practise calm breathing, when I'm beginning to feel stressed, like when I'm stuck in traffic en route to work. If I can't close my eyes and visualise, I find simply thinking about breathing in clean, nutritious oxygen and breathing out all fear and tension really helpful. The more you do it in these normal daily situations the more your brain and body get used to it. Generally, you start to feel calmer in stressful or difficult situations.

DOWN-BREATHING

Down-breathing is a slight switch in breathing technique for the pushing or second stage of labour. When you're fully dilated and feel the need to push we consider that to be the second stage of labour. (See page 199 for more on the stages and phases of labour.) You may feel a change of direction within your body and start to naturally feel 'pushy', as midwives say. You'll know when you need to switch breathing techniques.

This is about breathing with more intent and action behind it. You want to breathe in a little quicker through your nose and breathe out slowly with pure *downward* intent through your nose. You may also make some involuntary 'moo' sounds with this. Don't worry; that's a sign that your body is doing all the right things.

You may find that nose breathing goes out the window as you are pushing. You may want to control the breath through your nose but you just can't as your breathing changes with your body. If this is the case for you, breathe in any way that feels right. As long as you're focusing all your energy downwards.

A good time to practise this down-breathing is on the loo, especially if you have constipation. Try not to force or push while you're doing this; you want to breathe in and breathe out with focused downward intent. It's more of a mental process of directing your breath downwards.

This can be a little more difficult than the up breathing for some, because there's no counting involved, but once you've given it a go on the loo you should soon get the hang of it and may be surprised at how well downward breathing helps constipation.

Try to add visualisations to down-breathing too.

- Imagine opening like layers of a rose bud, gently and softly unfolding and opening with ease. This can help you imagine or visualise opening and creating space for your baby.

- Visualise a sensation or intention of a dropping of the pelvis towards the ground, while allowing anything above your pelvis to float upwards towards the sky to assist gravity to do its job. Rather than thinking of 'forcing' your baby out, imagine an expanding opening for your baby to navigate and exit their way out into the outside world.

RELAXATION FOR EVERY BIRTH

You don't need a particular set of circumstances to be able to get into a calm and relaxed state when you have practised and trained your brain. I have looked after women who have needed an emergency C-section and used hypnobirthing. One woman told me that while she was lying on the operating table waiting for the obstetrician, in her mind, by using breathing and visualisation, she was relaxing under a tree. She felt much calmer for being able to do this. So many mums have said that they don't know what they would have done without hypnobirthing during their labour and birth.

If your circumstances change in labour, the best thing you can do is accept the change of course. If you have considered risks (if there are any), looked at alternative options, considered what your gut instinct has told you, then now is the time to accept that you are where you are. I'm not suggesting you sit back and don't participate in your care. What I am suggesting is that you get comfortable with your individual risks, and what is currently available to you, so you can *move forward* rather than over-think and perhaps become overwhelmed or feel out of control.

No matter what type of birth you are planning or end up with, practising relaxation and breathing during pregnancy, birth and shortly after you have had your baby may help you better manage your emotions and your body's response to the changes you are experiencing.

KEY POINTS

- Aim to avoid engaging the thinking part of the brain (neocortex) during labour.
- The fetus ejection reflex means the body can give birth without any conscious thinking. When the mind is relaxed the body can get on with what it needs to.
- 'Letting go' allows the mammalian brain to take over and for the body to release the right hormones.
- Breathing techniques will help you get into a state of relaxation. You need to practise breathing and relaxation techniques daily to really reap the benefits.
- You can use hypnobirthing in any birth context.

How to choose your tribe

NOW YOU'VE GOT your toolkit ready, understand your birthing body and know how to get into a state of relaxation, it is time to think about your birth tribe. We are going to think about who you want at the birth, and what they need to do during the birth to make sure you get the best birth for you on the day.

CHOOSE YOUR TRIBE

Numbers wise, if you're having a baby in hospital you can have two people at your side, but if you're having a home birth you can have whoever you want (including the dog). As long as the midwife can safely and easily move around, the number is up to you.

Your chosen 'tribe,' a.k.a. birth partner(s), are key to having a positive birth experience and keeping your oxytocin levels flowing. As you now know, oxytocin is easily scared away, so your tribe need to be able to encourage your body to produce natural oxytocin and keep away the fear responses that reduce it.

Labour is like a marathon. Imagine you're running one, you're a fair way through and you're getting a little tired. No one is really supporting you, helping you stay on track or handing you drinks as you run past. How far would you get? Now imagine you're running a marathon and you've got people you love and trust supporting you, keeping you well hydrated, attending to your needs, supporting you each stride of your run, keeping you focused on the finish line. Now how far would you get? Your tribe should help you get to the finish line.

They should understand, support, guide and care for you. No one should be there for their own benefit; their presence must *only* benefit you. You need to be able to really trust your tribe so that you can completely let go of everything going on around you to focus on your breathing, relaxation, visualisations or simply resting between contractions. I've seen labours slow down significantly, and even stop after new members of 'the tribe' have joined. Once a woman's mother-in-law went to get food after her labour was starting to slow down. After her mother-in-law left, the woman changed position and gave birth about 20 minutes later. It could be coincidence but it's not the first time I have seen a labour totally turn around after a change in company.

Energy around birth needs to be slow and accepting. Most people have a focus on wanting the baby out, which is perfectly understandable. It's hard not to look forward to that incredible moment but the drive to want that can change the atmosphere (remember your oxytocin enhancers, page 176). We've all been sat next to or near someone who is stressed, and you can almost see and feel it oozing out of them. Tone of voice can even have an impact; you can hear the stress in someone's tone of voice, especially if you know them well. Tone of voice is thought to affect the physiology of the body and the physiological process of labour is vulnerable to interruption, so let your tribe know this before labour. If you know someone isn't good at keeping chilled and calm in a emotionally charged situation, then perhaps they are not the right person to be with you during birth.

SHOULD YOUR PARTNER BE PRESENT AT BIRTH?

People say different things about having men at birth. Deborah Lewis, the first Vice-President of the International Confederation of Midwives from the Caribbean, explains in her TED Talk that fathers should be at the birth of their child because families thrive when fathers are present at birth, and their involvement, engagement and support is critical. She says that being present at the birth kick-starts the nurturing instinct for fathers, and highlights that when fathers are involved in preparation for birth and decision-making there are fewer complications and interventions for women. Your partner usually knows about your body and behaviour in a way that nobody else does, so this does make sense.

It is believed that the male hormonal composition changes during labour. Testosterone is thought to drop and men release a surge of oxytocin at birth, which helps initiate bonding.

However, Michel Odent (obstetrician and childbirth specialist) thinks that having a male partner at a birth can slow progress. He believes that having the partner present is a new phenomenon and in the animal kingdom, female mammals give birth alone, away from their sexual partner. He feels that since the mid nineteenth century, the maternity environment has become masculinised and he thinks this may interfere with the mother's natural processes, such as being protective. The maternal protective-aggressive instinct that occurs directly after birth – it is the moment when a woman is at her most powerful (imagine a gorilla protecting her newborn!). And yet, by 'socialising' birth, Odent argues, humanity has neutralised this force.

Another consideration is: how does your partner feel about being there? My friend's partner categorically stated, that he did not, under any circumstances, want to be present at the birth of any of his four children. He is a perfectly good father and husband: he changed nappies, pushed prams, cooked, and treated the boys and girls with equality, but he didn't want to be at the birth. So he wasn't. His wife respected his decision and was happy for him not to be there. If someone is at your birth who doesn't really want to be or feels frightened, then all this will do is add stress and pressure to the situation. Whether your partner is male or female it doesn't matter. They may not feel comfortable being at your birth. Sometimes these feelings can come from not wanting to see you in pain or not wanting to see you and your body in a non-sexual way. It is controversial but worth considering if your partner wants to be there or not.

If they do not want to be there perhaps talk about their reasons why and then consider who you would like instead. A woman who has had a baby herself, whether that is a mum or friend, can be really helpful and reassuring. We'll go on to talk about the power of doulas in a minute too.

You know what is best for you, your body and your relationship. I don't believe it is our place as healthcare professionals to advise you whether to have your partner with you or not; it is, again, your choice. This section focuses on what I know about birth partners, (whether they are the partner/father or not), their role and how they can really help or hinder birth.

IF YOUR NAME'S NOT ON THE LIST, YOU'RE NOT COMING IN

When helping women decide who they're going to ask to be at their birth, I ask them to think about people they'd feel least embarrassed walking in on them having sex! Never an ideal scenario, but really think about this when you go through each person you think you might want at your birth. I have a few people I'm close to and we'd laugh it off, and then there's others who would be utterly *horrified*. Sometimes, the people in the latter group make their way into a woman's birth. This can really slow birth down; the human brain takes over and you think you should, or are in some way obliged to, let them observe your birth. Telling your partner and any key people who you are having at the birth now might be awkward, but your birth is not a spectacle and it is not about what other people want. Birth is a major life event, and it should be kept as private and undisturbed as possible, so we need to protect your space surrounding it.

WHY YOUR TRIBE MATTERS

Having good support has been widely studied, and it has been found that continuous support reduced labour length, reduced birth analgesia and also increased spontaneous vaginal delivery. A Cochrane study states:

'We found 26 studies that provided data from 17 countries, involving more than 15,000 women in a wide range of settings and circumstances. The continuous support was provided either by hospital staff (such as nurses or midwives), or women who were not hospital employees and had no personal relationship to the labouring woman (such as doulas or women who were provided with a modest amount of guidance on providing support). In other cases, the support came from companions of the woman's choice from her own network (such as her partner, mother, or friend).

'Women who received continuous labour support may be more likely to give birth 'spontaneously', i.e. give birth vaginally with neither ventouse nor forceps nor Caesarean. In addition, women may be less likely to use pain medications or to have a Caesarean birth, and may be more likely to be satisfied and have shorter labours. Postpartum depression could be lower in women who were supported in labour, but we cannot be sure of this due to the studies being difficult to compare (they were in different settings, with different people giving support). The babies of women who received continuous support may be less likely to have low five-minute Apgar scores (the score used when babies' health and well-being are assessed at birth and shortly afterwards).'

If supportive birth partners were a drug, every woman would be recommended to take it.

Here are some of the main 'jobs' of your tribe as I see it:

- To look after your emotional wellbeing, and to make sure you feel safe and cared for. They need to offer kind words of support and encouragement.
- To follow your lead. You may ask for different things when you are in labour and if this happens your birth tribe needs to have your back. They need to adapt to your changing needs. For example, in the latent phase (see page 200) you may want more touch and words of encouragement but if you're in 'the zone' further along in labour you may not want any touching, only minimal talking and to go deep within yourself. Changes in your needs are normal and your tribe need to be able to adapt and accept this.
- To know your plans and preferences so they are fully on board with everything and can calmly relay your plan or answer any questions if you're in 'labour land'. They are your voice, echoing exactly what you want and acting for you when you need them to. They also need to be

good communicators and create an atmosphere of teamwork. Often a birth partner will want to fix things but it is good to let them know that there is nothing to fix and that this is a normal and natural process. If they are up for it, ask them to join you in watching videos of positive births. They need to see and also trust the birth process. If you are getting tired and a little self-doubt is creeping in, it is your tribe that will help hold you up and keep you going.

- To help you with breathing and relaxation techniques if you would like them to. Your birth partner needs to know about the oxytocin enhancers (see page 176) and how to keep your oxytocin flowing. Some romantic partners cuddle, have a little kiss and hold hands throughout labour. Others don't feel like doing this or aren't in a romantic relationship and opt for massages or gentle stroking instead.
- To offer practical support to make the plan happen. For example, if you want a home water birth, then they need to know how to assemble and fill the pool. If driving you to hospital, they need to have change in the car for the car park or make sure you have easy access to transport in labour. Throughout labour, they should also make sure you are well hydrated (this really helps your uterus muscle perform at its best), have the right music/hypnobirthing track playing, keep the room as dimly lit and quiet as possible, and if you are having a homebirth they need to get the towels at the ready. Also make sure the midwives know where the kettle is!

What to do if there's nothing to do

Sometimes in labour your birth partner(s) are unsure about what they can do because the truth is, at times during birth there isn't a lot for them to do. Which is why the media need to add their take on birth and over-dramatise it. Sometimes I barely do anything at birth other than my clinical observations and interject if it's needed. When it comes to your tribe, they need to know that just their presence, calmness and patience is all that you may need and it is okay to 'do nothing' – they aren't a spare part; they are still supporting you by just being there. Their trusted presence influences your mindset. That's why if ever there's a formal investigation at a work place, you can bring someone for support. Going into a meeting or investigation is a lot easier if you have someone with you, even if they don't say a word.

You may also want to tell your birth partner, that it's okay for them to go and have a snooze, a cuppa or eat something when you don't fancy eating. I have seen many birth partners struggling to keep their eyes open and the birthing woman is perfectly happy doing her own thing; the birth partner could be having a snooze or getting some snacks in. She really wouldn't mind but they don't know that so they sit there struggling – just to be on the safe side. Or perhaps you want the opposite; you might want to know your birth partners are there with you every minute of your labour. Whatever it is, let them know what you prefer so they don't disturb you asking or sit there hungry and bleary-eyed.

Lastly, you may want to delegate someone to take photos, unless you chose to hire a birth photographer. Have a think about who's going to be taking photos in those precious moments.

A NOTE TO BIRTH PARTNERS

If you are expecting your first baby or have been asked to be a birth partner then I'm sure you are nervous, excited and perhaps not quite sure what to expect or what is expected of you. Here's the heads-up on what to expect and some handy tips.

- **We are here for you too.** If you are worried about something, have a question for your midwife or a particular wish, just let us know. Primarily, midwives and doctors will focus on the woman and the baby during labour and birth but if you need something, please let them know. You really matter too and midwives are happy to answer questions and make sure you have a positive birth experience too.
- **You may need a break.** As labour progresses, emotions can run high but you really need to look after yourself as both mum and baby will need your support after birth. First babies can take their time and even if your partner can't eat, have a snack and keep yourself hydrated – you need to look after yourself too. If you are not sure if this is the right time to go for a break, ask her and/or the midwife.
- **Your emotions will be running high.** You may be intensely needed or not, you may feel helpless, excited, nervous and even

uncomfortable. You may need to rely on healthcare professionals to look after your partner and your baby. As these emotions arise, try to stay as calm and relaxed as possible. It is important to be patient when it comes to birth. Asking things like 'how much longer will it be?' can (totally innocently) create a time pressure for her. If things need to move along, midwives or doctors will usually recommend intervention. Otherwise, it is best to assume everything is unfolding naturally and normally.

- **Your support is so important.** It can be hard to know how the woman is as she may not want to talk or be her usual self. Try not to ask her questions (unless you really need to) but offer words of encouragement instead. Being sensitive to her changing needs will go a long way. It is normal for women to want one thing one minute, and then absolutely not want it the next minute; you're not doing anything wrong – things have just changed. If you are together as a couple you are setting the foundations for your new family and she'll remember your help forever. Don't underestimate how important your hand-holding and trust in her really is.

- **Go through the labour bag.** It will most likely be you that has to grab bits and bobs from the labour bag whilst she is in labour, so make sure you know where everything is so you haven't got to pull it all out when either of you needs something quickly. If you're having a homebirth, have a little area for the things she might ask for, like lip balm or a hair tie. You also need to make sure you've got drinks at the ready for both of you. Women easily get dehydrated in labour, especially if they are in a pool. The room is usually kept warm for when baby arrives, so you may get dehydrated too. I usually ask birth partners to look after the drinks, making sure they are flowing (unless a drip is being used).

Remember, if she has asked you to be there, she really trusts you and I'm sure you will be an amazing birth partner. Don't underestimate yourself!

WHAT ABOUT DOULAS?

The easiest way to explain the difference between a midwife and a doula is that a midwife is a healthcare provider and a doula is more of a birth companion. A doula is trained in supporting women before, during and after birth. They impart their knowledge, confidence and experience of birth through helping with change of position, massage, words of encouragement, support and much more. They are not medically trained, cannot give medication, do observations or carry out any tests. A doula is there solely to help and support you emotionally and physically and they cannot replace a midwife. Their care usually starts in pregnancy and they will get to know you throughout your journey to ensure they only drive your agenda. After the birth, most doulas also provide one or two postnatal visits in order to answer any questions, debrief the birth and support you with feeding your baby. These postnatal visits are really helpful to women too.

Trained doulas have been clinically proven to reduce the length of labour, lead to less intervention and more positive memories of birth. They are also known to help fathers take on their new role with confidence, increase success in breastfeeding and decrease risk of postnatal depression. How do they create such magic? Because your doula knows your plans, your parameters and your preferences. She is only there for you and to support you emotionally. Even if you have a supportive partner, best friend, mother or sister, still consider a doula.

> 'If a woman doesn't look like a Goddess in labour, someone isn't doing their job right'
>
> **— INA MAY GASKIN**

When it comes to hiring a doula, it's about finding the right doula for you and your family. It is important we all work together as a team – partners, midwives, doulas and doctors – because we all want to achieve the same goal. We need to respect the vital roles we all play during birth and it is important we all know when to act and when to sit back. Overall, I have had brilliant experiences with doulas and the team work has been on point. To ensure this feeling of team work is brought into your birth it might be a good idea to introduce your doula to your midwife or doctor. Even if that is just at one of your regular antenatal appointments so that they can all meet and ensure that you get the best possible care from your birth team.

A good place to search for a doula is Doula UK; it is the largest voluntary organisation representing doulas in the UK. Each doula operates independently, but in order to join they will have had to attend a Doula UK approved preparation course and abide by the organisation's strict code of conduct.

It's not realistic for everyone to be able to afford a doula, especially when you have to buy other products for your baby or are living off a single income. If you would really like to hire a doula, but would struggle to pay their usual fees, it is always worth getting in touch and having a chat with them. A lot of doulas are willing to offer payment plans, negotiate reduced fees if you are in real financial need, or they may be interested in an exchange of services or goods instead of cash.

You can get Doula UK gift vouchers to offset some of the cost of hiring a doula. If people are going to buy you something anyway, you may as well get something that could really impact your whole birth experience. Most people don't know what to buy pregnant women so they'll opt for babywear or a cuddly toy but there's no harm in being honest and saying what you want.

'I COULDN'T HAVE DONE IT WITHOUT THEM'

Although this is not actual scientific research, over the years and during my travels around the world, I have asked women about their birth experience, both when things went according to plan and when they didn't. The same phrases kept popping up and still do now. Those who had good support usually start with focusing on the help and support they had saying things like, 'I couldn't have done it without them' and even when an emergency situation has occurred they are more positive and accepting. The company and support at birth has such an impact on the physiology of the labouring body. You need to really trust, feel comfortable and connect with your midwife, and it is perfectly okay to request a different midwife if you need to. Your birth partner can approach this if you don't want to or are in the zone, either way, speaking up about how someone is making you feel is so important. This is one of the biggest moments of your life and you don't have to have someone there who isn't making you feel comfortable (although this is extremely rare). It is your body, your baby, your birth and your decision. You're the boss in the birth room. Whether women have their perfect birth or an unplanned intervention it is the support that really stands out.

KEY POINTS

- Choose your tribe wisely – they need to protect your environment and help you feel calm.
- Natural oxytocin is released when we feel happy, loved and safe – your birth tribe are partly responsible for this.
- Plan your birth with your birth partner.
- Sometimes the presence and support is all you need; your birth partner doesn't always have to be busy.
- Birth companions reduce the length of labour, the need for analgesia and lead to more positive feelings about birth.
- Consider a doula and ask for gift vouchers if you're on a budget.

Giving birth: it's not a race

NOW YOU UNDERSTAND how labour works and have your support team in place, it's time to go onto the stages of labour, what to expect, and how to manage your own labour.

THE STAGES OF LABOUR

You might have heard about the different stages of labour before. They can be a little confusing as some talk about 'early', 'latent', 'active', 'first stage', 'pushing stage', etc. According to our midwife training, there are three stages of labour:

- The first stage is where your uterus is contracting, causing your cervix to dilate enough for your baby to pass through (about 10cm). We also call this 'established' labour.
- The second stage is where you push your baby out.
- The third stage is when you deliver your placenta.

In reality there is a lot more to labour than that. The three stages misses out a few phases of labour that women and midwives tend to refer to more often so we will go over those too. You probably won't really know or care much about the various stages at the time, and to be honest you don't really need to focus on stages or centimetres. They may all merge into one or you may be able to tell them apart when you're there. Either way, you need to know what to expect and what it feels like so you can go with your labouring body and trust the process.

First stage: Latent labour

Another phase to think about is the time before you are in the established part of labour. This is the very beginning of labour, where you'll have *that* thought ('I think something is happening . . .'). If you are more than 37 weeks pregnant you are considered to be 'full term' and if labour starts, it might not be quite what you were expecting, but it's okay. Your baby is mature enough to come out. Early labour can feel like period pain; it is a crampy sensation and your tummy starts going tight but it is different to the Braxton Hicks you may have been having.

The cramps can start to radiate around your back or start in your back and radiate around to the front. They are usually fairly short-lasting and don't have a real pattern to them yet. Some women also get pain down their thighs with the tightenings. You will most likely be able to talk during this stage at first, but as it progresses, and contractions get closer, you'll gradually need to stop and start to breathe your way through (see page 183). You may also lose your 'mucus plug' (the protective barrier). Appearance-wise, it can look a bit snotty and might be slightly blood-stained. It's not quite the knight in shining armour, but none the less, it has done a marvellous job of protecting your baby. Your waters may or may not go at this stage. Some women are really surprised at the amount of water there is; it can be way more than you think and it will carry on leaking out until you have your baby. If you think they have gone you need to give your midwife a call and let her know. She'll do a quick assessment and if everything is normal, your baby is moving, the fluid is clear (with no signs of meconium which is brown or green), no smell and you have no further complications (or known Group B strep) then usually we don't need to do anything. You can just wait for your labour to progress naturally, but this is unique to each individual so you need to discuss this with your midwife.

A NOTE ON GROUP B STREP

Before getting your own home testing for GBS it is so important that you are fully informed about GBS and not misled by media stories or individual experiences. Dr Sara Wickam has an up-to-date, evidence-based short book and free articles on her website, about GBS.

You might hear the word 'niggling' being used; midwives love the word and often use it to describe the start of the latent phase of labour. I don't know where it comes from but it is a well-known international term that we use. Niggling usually means you are getting short, irregular contractions, maybe one every 15–20 minutes or even one every 10 minutes but they don't last long or have any predictable pattern.

The latent (or 'niggling') phase generally doesn't mean you're about to have your baby. I have never seen a baby born with contractions that are 10–15 minutes apart and that are short-lasting. It has probably happened somewhere in the world (there are always exceptions) but it is pretty much unheard of, especially with first babies.

You don't need to call your midwife if you are in latent phase and your waters have not gone yet. The exception is if you have a planned C-section or have been advised to call her for any other reason. Some community or independent midwives may like to know that something is starting so they have a bit more warning, but otherwise midwives don't generally need to know yet. The best place for you to be is in the comfort of your own home, and your body will progress faster at home during this phase.

That said, there are some circumstances where home may not be the best place for you. If you do not feel safe at home, don't feel like you can cope with the contractions, or are alone and need support then call the midwife as soon as you need to. Don't feel like you *have* to wait.

You can call your midwife any time you like, but you really need to if:

- Your baby's movements have changed.
- What's coming out is not the mucus plug or you are bleeding.
- You need pain relief or are not getting any breaks between contractions.
- You have been in latent phase all day/night and do not feel anything is progressing.
- You are concerned about anything or have a question – we're here for you.

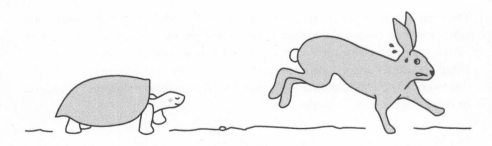

HOW TO BE A TORTOISE

Labour could be the biggest endurance challenge your body will face so you need to *take it slow*. Imagine you have a marathon to run, so now is the time to conserve energy and pace yourself. Getting to the finish line is the top priority and running out of resources may jeopardise this. Sometimes women go for long walks, start moving the furniture, pulling the cot around and go into action mode in early labour. By the time they are ready to give birth they're shattered. There's some advice floating around that offers early labour activities like baking cakes and walking up and down stairs. Ignore it. If you start doing these you're spending your limited resources unnecessarily. If you feel like doing some gentle yoga, hip openers or squatting that's fine, but overall it is best to conserve your energy, relax and be gentle on yourself.

Most women spend the majority of labour in the latent phase, as the cervix needs to soften, come forward and dilate, so there is plenty going on. To feel an example of how your cervix changes, touch the end of your nose; fairly firm isn't it? Now touch your lips, quite a difference, isn't there? They're softer and easier to move. Your nose feels more like a non-labouring cervix and an established labouring cervix feels more like your lips. The cervix needs to go from firm and closed to softer, stretcher and open by 4–5cm. That difference means your body has to go through quite a lot of change; your cervix has been shut, firmly holding your baby in and your uterus has been relaxed, allowing your baby to grow and your tummy to expand. Now your cervix needs to relax and open, and your uterus needs to tighten to push your baby down. They know what they need to do; they just need a little time to switch over and get going. Like when a DJ suddenly changes the tunes from slow jams to club music, it can sometimes take a while to adjust to the new rhythm and bust out the most appropriate dance moves ...

RELAXING IN THE LATENT PHASE

'The latent phase can sometimes be long and drawn-out, and it can be easy to forget that this can be normal. In the weeks before baby's arrival, make a little place in your home that is your "safe place". Each day go to this place and play the same piece of music, have the same fragrant candle/oil smell (lavender is perfect) and spend 10 minutes or so just visualising on baby and making a connection. Then, if your labour is stopping and starting and you are dealing with contractions at home, you can go to your "safe place" to re-focus and ground yourself when you feel you are not coping and losing your focus.'

Samantha Pantlin, *The Naked Midwives*

Sometimes this stage can be a bit stop-start, so you think 'ahh this is it ...' then it all stops before picking up again. Although everyone is different, if you suspect you have been in the latent phase all day, and haven't yet told your midwife or doctor, I would recommend you let someone know and always make sure you are still happy with your baby's movements.

Relaxing can sometimes be hard if labour doesn't start or progress as quickly as you'd like, I know. But when you get frustrated or anxious in labour, you start to change your birth biology and create mixed messages leading to uncertainty. As you know from 'Step out of the way and trust your body' (see page 173) this is because your body and uterus are protective. If you start to feel anxious it is translated to your uterus as, 'I'm not sure the outside world is safe right now. Best to keep baby in here.'

To help turn this around and send the 'It's safe to come out now' message, try putting your attention onto any feeling of frustration. Observe it fully; where are you feeling it the most? Your mind? Maybe deep in the pit of your stomach? Try to identify where it is coming from. Take a deep breath in, and as you breathe out, let your shoulders drop and let those feelings of frustration go. You may need a few breaths to let it all go. Once the frustration has been released, turn your attention to focus on the fact your body doing its very best, your body is so clever, protective and able. You've got this.

EARLY LABOUR TO-DO LIST

If you're like me and always need a to-do list, even when there's nothing to *do*, here's some suggestions:

- Listen to your tracks if you are hypnobirthing and start using your techniques.
- Watch a funny film or TV series.
- Ask your birth partner for a gentle foot rub.
- Have a candlelit bath with a drop of lavender oil in it, or sit in the shower and let the lovely warm water wash over you.
- Meditate or try some simple yoga.
- Have a little bounce on your birth ball.
- Lie down on your side, put a pillow between your legs, breathe deep and doze if you can.
- Get going on the snacks, whatever you fancy, and start to sip water ... you'll need to be well hydrated.

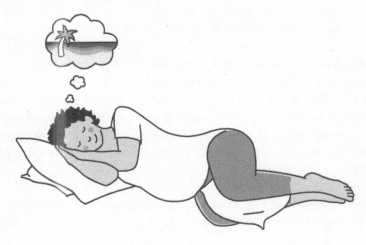

LABOUR HYDRATION AND FUEL

Dehydration can cause complications in labour. Many women that come into hospital for labour assessments are already dehydrated (we can tell from the urine dip and a fast heart rate, among other things), and this can sometimes cause the baby to have a slightly higher heart rate; in this case we will recommend a CTG monitoring (a 20-minute monitoring of your baby's heart rate.) The good news is dehydration is easily preventable by drinking water little and often; drink whenever you feel thirsty and make sure water is within your reach. You may need more if you are immersed in warm water. You can give the 'drink job' to your birth partner, if you like, and ask them to make sure they keep the drinks flowing. It is also important for you to keep peeing too because an empty bladder will help create more room for your baby's head to come down through your pelvis.

Blood sugar can also drop in labour and this can then slow labour down, so eat little and often if you can. Have whatever you fancy, but most women don't feel like eating a full meal so snacks like natural fruit and grain bars, nuts, crackers, flapjacks, dates and fruit are good to keep sugar levels up and keep you going. Some women like to have little teaspoons or licks of honey. Whatever floats your boat; as long as you are getting something in while you can because you probably won't feel like eating in the next phase of labour.

Note: Diabetic women, this may be different for you – stick to the dietary advice your specialist midwife has given you.

USE YOUR BIRTHING BALL

When you are crossing over from latent to established labour it can be a struggle to get comfy in any position but if you are familiar with your ball positions and have been experimenting in pregnancy you should be able to get into a comfortable place and be able to release tension in your lower back. Your pelvic floor has already been under strain during pregnancy but a ball provides soft and gentle support for it too. While you're on the ball you naturally assume positions that encourage your baby to get into a good position down in your pelvis too – those upright, forward and open (UFO) positions. Sometimes women end up with sore wrists as they've put a lot of weight on them by pushing against or leaning on hard surfaces, so be mindful not to place too much strain on your wrists.

First stage: Established labour

This is when you need to have a midwife care for you. You need to call your midwife when your contractions have established a nice regular pattern, usually about three contractions in a ten-minute period (3:10), each lasting about 45 seconds.

You will probably feel like things have started to 'ramp up' in this stage. If this is not your first baby you should call your midwife before they are 3:10; you know your body so use your judgement here and call if you think your labour is establishing. Labour can progress more quickly if your body has done it before.

When you arrive at hospital or the MLU, or if your midwife comes out to you at home, you will be offered a vaginal examination to see how far dilated your cervix is, this is called a 'labour assessment'. According to national maternity guidelines, you are considered to be in established labour when your cervix is 4–5cm dilated or more and you are having strong, regular contractions.

Your definition of your own labour may be different to ours, and that doesn't mean you are wrong if you feel like you are in established labour but your cervix is less than 4cm. So that hospitals and midwives can make sure that women, who are expected to have their baby soon, receive one-to-one care, it is necessary to have these *guidelines* to go by. If you feel like things are progressing faster or you need pain relief then let us know – you are at the centre of your own care.

When you have turned your neocortex down, you'll be 'more primal' and less communicative, and this is fine! Midwives see women come into hospital or the MLU in all different ways; whether you are silent and still, or louder, making funny noises, and leaking amniotic fluid, it really doesn't matter. What matters is knowing how to stay in-tune with your primal self. Everything we have gone through so far, like your toolkit, breathing and relaxation and your birth partners, can help you do this.

It is standard practice for midwives to offer routine vaginal examinations once labour has established; this is to assess how your labour is progressing. You do not have to have *any* examinations if you don't want to, you can just have the initial assessment or you can have them every four hours. The choice is yours. If you are unsure, your midwife will be able to help you make this choice at the time, especially if your dilation would gain valuable information or effect a decision that you need to make.

Things tend to speed up a little bit in this stage – you can be in latent phase for a long time (which is why you need to be a tortoise) but once you have lasting, regular contractions, your cervix *tends* to dilate quicker – mainly if you are in the right environment, are moving and changing positions, with the right support, and feel safe. It's now that you will really need your oxytocin enhancers to help your labour progress. Head back to page 176 for a recap. In short, this is the time to be drawing the curtains, getting out the essential oils, be more active (if you feel like it) and putting your labour music/hypnobirthing tracks on.

If you are planning a water birth and feel like getting in the pool, then now is the time to go for it. Water can be such a lovely release and you can also get into different positions you may not normally be able to; the buoyancy gives you more freedom to move. You can also rest more during the breaks between contractions because you don't need to support your body as much.

Gravity is your friend. If you are still mobile and are not getting in a pool then the more upright you are the better – gravity really helps you out by putting pressure on your cervix so it continues to dilate beautifully. Bean bags also are brilliant because they adapt and fit around you to help support your body. And keep using your birthing ball, if you like.

If you have had an epidural, you still have options to help things along, like going on your side or sitting upright. Some hospitals have invested in funky beds, which help you get into a seated position with your legs lowered. If you have allowed the epidural to wear off a bit (which can sometimes be advised just before pushing) you may be able to go onto all-fours supported by the bed before you start pushing. Although TV shows would suggest that lying on your back is the usual way to give birth, it can stop gravity helping you. If you're lying down on your back it creates an upward curve for your pelvis, meaning

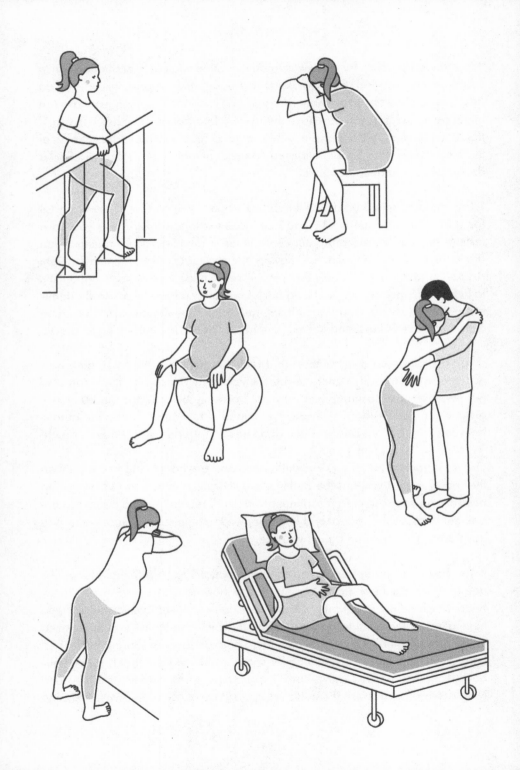

your baby needs to come up over your pelvis; if you are more upright and open, your baby can come down into your pelvis easier.

If you need a CTG (continuous cardiotocography, the electronic monitoring of your baby's heartrate) you can still be mobile or use your ball and you don't have to lie on a bed.

As established labour progresses, most women start to go into themselves and can't or don't feel like talking anymore.

First stage: Transition
Transition is when your cervix is almost fully dilated (10cm) and you are nearly ready to start pushing. Sometimes your contractions will space out a little bit too. There is a distinct feeling at this stage; many women have a moment of self-doubt, an overwhelming feeling of irritability and even a little panic. It is okay to feel all of those things. It is the shift of power within the body that is making you stop and feel like that. You are there. Right up on the finish line, about to meet your baby. The feeling is intense, but short-lived. If you have had an epidural you may not feel this, but don't worry; it is all happening as it should and your midwife will help to guide you when is time to push.

My friend, who is a midwife, knew she was in transition, but even so, the feelings took over, just for a moment. She said: 'I know I am in transition, but I just want to go home now. I can't do it! Can I just go home?' Ten minutes later she had her baby in her arms. Just keep going – your midwife and your birth partner will be right there with you supporting you and encouraging you.

Second stage: Pushing
This is the labour stage that most of us talk, think and hear about so it may come as a surprise that this stage is usually shorter than the latent and established phases of labour. It's a common misconception that labour is all about pushing. Everyone is different but what is mostly the same is how you feel at this stage. You'll naturally start feel the urge to push (like you need a big poo!), or you might start to make involuntary sounds, grunting or sometimes a full-on moo. These are all totally normal signs that you are ready to start pushing. Many women like the pushing stage, mostly because they are able to really use their contractions and take on an active role. Not to mention the excitement – you are about to meet your baby!

No matter where you are, whether you have an epidural or not, it is important to get into a position that is most comfortable for you and as upright as possible or on all-fours. If you don't have an epidural and are using hypnobirthing you may want to go with your body and prefer not to be guided on pushing. However, some women want their midwife to talk them through this stage. Whatever you choose, it is important to give your perineum time to stretch and slow the speed of your baby's head crowning, so let's go over that now.

Most often midwives recommend you pant. This kind of breathing encourages tiny, gentle, slower movements rather than rapid force and quick progression. If women need me to help guide them through this stage, and the head is crowning, I usually advise women to breathe like they are blowing out candles on a birthday cake. My dad is a driving instructor and he often tells his pupils 'less space, less speed'. If you go flying down a road with little space either side of your car you are more likely to damage the car. But, if you take it easy and go slow you'll probably get fewer scratches. This is a similar concept with birth, but with the added ability of your vagina to change shape (unlike the road). Your body can sometimes take over and just push, and the burning sensation caused by stretching can get intense, but this is where your perineal massaging will pay off. You will have built up a bit of a tolerance and prepared your skin to stretch that little bit more. If you're not in the water this is when your midwife can apply the warm pack (see page 124). Trust guidelines vary around the country for the expected time it takes to push a baby out but NICE state the expected time is up to three hours from the start of active pushing if it is your first baby, and within two hours for most women who have had a baby before. This stage is the most triumphant of all. You get to meet, cuddle and explore your little baby!

Third stage: Nearly there!
The last thing to do is to deliver the placenta. As badass and hardcore as the placenta is when your baby is growing, it is soft in texture and far easier to deliver. It is about the size of a small pizza (depending on where you get your take-aways from). Your midwife will talk you through everything and explain what is happening. If you have chosen to have the injection for your placenta it will be given in your upper thigh just after your baby is born. The injection helps your uterus to contract down and expel the placenta and reduces initial blood loss, but it can make you feel sick. Some women prefer not to have this unless they are at risk of bleeding. Your midwife will be able to advise you on what is safest for you and you can make an informed choice (see page 100).

Sometimes before the placenta comes out there is a separation bleed. This can look a bit scary and as though you are bleeding fairly heavily, but don't worry, it is normal and should stop by itself. Usually the separation bleed is a sign the placenta has come away from your uterus and that is what has caused the bleed. All those blood vessels that have been pumping blood to your baby need to constrict and close over. If this bleed goes on for longer than expected your midwife may recommend you have the injection (or a second dose if you have had one) alongside some other intervention and drugs to stop further bleeding.

THE BEST TIME TO CUT THE CORD

When your baby is born it will be attached to you via the umbilical cord, which is attached to the placenta. About one-third of your baby's blood volume is still circulating in the cord and placenta. In the minutes following the birth this blood is still rich with iron, oxygen and stem cells; an impressive combination in terms of our biology. A cord with blood in it is fat, full and sort of bluish in colour – if we cut the cord when it's like this then we are potentially depriving your baby of that extra goodness. If possible, it is best to 'wait for white', so your baby can get the full transfusion of rich blood. This means, quite literally, waiting for the cord to turn white and therefore has emptied itself of blood before it is cut. This takes around five minutes after the birth of a baby.

If for whatever reason it is not possible to wait for white, national guidelines state a minimum delay of one minute for all births, unless there is a concern over the ability of the cord or the baby's heartbeat.

A PLANNED C-SECTION

If you have a planned section it is unlikely that you will experience any of the stages of labour, although you might get a few 'niggles' before the planned day. In the days or hours leading up to your section you may start to get a little nervous; don't worry, almost all the women I have looked after with a planned section feel the build-up of nerves. Remember that even though you are having an operation and are perhaps slightly more reliant on the hospital staff, you are still very much in control of what happens. You can still use all the hypnobirthing and breathing techniques you have learned, and you can still have many of your plans met, like delayed cord clamping, skin-to-skin and opting for a gentle or 'woman-centred' Caesarean section (see page 103). Your birth partner and midwife will be there to support you and ask all the questions you need to every step of the way.

USE YOUR BRAIN TOOL

Every woman, birth and baby are different. Sometimes babies get distressed in labour and this is shown through things like a change in baby's heart rate or thick meconium, which will come out in your waters (where baby has done a poo inside). These things are unpredictable. You can follow the best advice and do everything in your power to have a natural birth but last-minute changes can still happen. Remember that you *always* have your BRAIN tool (see page 37). If things change, try to remain calm and focused; it is rare that the situation is a true emergency. More often than not you have time to go through your options and make the best decision for you and your baby at the time. Your midwife and doctor will support you through any unexpected changes – everything is still a choice.

KEY POINTS

- The latent phase of labour is usually the longest phase.
- Slow and steady wins the race. Don't bake cakes and rush around; save your energy for when it's most needed.
- If you are low risk, aren't planning a homebirth and do not have any concerns, try to stay at home as long as possible.
- Call you midwife anytime for anything – we're here for you.
- In established labour relax as much as possible, and stay upright to let gravity help relax your cervix.
- Keep your environment as relaxed as possible with your oxytocin enhancers.
- You've got this.

You're not the only one in labour: your baby is too

THE CLASSIC ANALOGY of 'being pushed through the eye of a needle' couldn't be further from the truth about birth. Your best birth partner is your baby. During labour you and your baby work together. In fact, since you started puberty and then through each menstrual cycle, your body has been preparing for pregnancy, and throughout pregnancy your body has been getting ready for birth. Your uterus, pelvis and baby all come together in a collective team-effort during labour.

Nevertheless, unsolicited comments like 'you look like you're ready to pop!' or the ultimate flattery, 'are you sure you're not having twins!?' can start to get in your head. The media don't exactly help with their horrifying headlines either such as 'woman gives birth to giant baby'. When you've got a good-sized bump, it makes this idea all the more realistic. Try to forget all this nonsense and look at the facts, biology and everything we have learnt so far. Know that your body is designed to do this and your baby is your best birth partner, and here's how.

Your baby has been well looked after, but they know when it is time to leave and are well prepared at term (from 37 weeks onwards). During labour there is an intricate process of communication between your body and your baby that no one truly understands ... yet.

What we do understand is that your baby's head is not a bowling ball. Not much of a spoiler alert, I know, but sometimes women imagine they need to push out this big hard head, but it's really not like that. I'm sure you've heard people talk about the 'soft spot' on a baby's head (the fontanelles). There are extra bones in the skull to allow baby's head to pass through your pelvis. We start off with around 300 bones at birth and by the time we're 25, we have around 206 as they fuse together. Although the head is bony, it's softer and can easily change shape – we call this 'moulding'.

When we do a vaginal examination, midwives and doctors feel for the fontanelles on a baby's head to determine the position of the baby. It sounds clever when we tell you 'your baby is looking over to your right' but it's actually not that difficult when you understand the fetal skull and feel for the little gaps between the bones. It is completely different to how an adult bone feels to touch. Lots of babies worry their parents (right from the start!) when they come out with elongated heads, but their heads soon go back to a more rounded-looking shape. This clever design allows your baby to work with you and your pelvis.

FETAL BRAIN AND SKULL BEFORE AND DURING LABOUR:

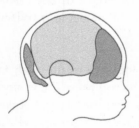
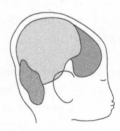

BEFORE LABOUR   **DURING LABOUR**

Skull shifting during birth has been happening in humans and their ancestors for millions of years because it's an adaptation to the evolution of larger brains and the change to upright walking, which in turn altered the shape of the pelvis. Incredible stuff!

The best position for your baby, ready for birth, is:

- Head down.
- Their back to your front – as though they are looking towards your spine.

- Their bum pushing forward.
- Their chin tucked in so the smallest part of their head is coming first.

Most babies will try to get into this position by themselves and if you have been a UFO (upright, forward and open) in pregnancy (see page 107) then this will really help your baby in labour and birth.

If you have a baby that is not in this position, there is some good advice on spinningbabies.com. If your baby is in the breech position (bottom down) your midwife will also discuss another option called ECV (external cephalic version) where an experienced doctor physically turns the baby around into a head-down position.

YOUR UTERUS IN ACTION

By the end of pregnancy, the purpose of your uterus is to empty itself. I know this may not be the emotional and beautiful explanation you expected, but it is the absolute truth. Your uterus has a specific job and it takes this job very seriously. It has been practising (as early as 24 weeks) for labour with Braxton Hicks. Your uterus has been stretched and provided your baby with a place to grow, but it has been preparing for the grand finale – labour and birth.

When I picture the job of the uterus, I imagine a dinner party I once hosted. Several people came over and I was so excited. I got everything prepared hours before and waited for their arrival. They took longer than I thought to show up but I was relieved when they did as I'd done so much preparation. I served them like I would royalty and did all the clearing up after them. We spent some real quality time together and had a lovely evening but as it drew to a close, I got tired and just wanted them to leave. We've all been there. It's all right when you're the one that can leave but when you're in your own home it's a game-changer. So, I did everything in my power to encourage and hint towards them leaving. I was talking about all the stuff I had to do the next day and how I just don't function well without a solid seven hours' sleep, all while looking at the clock ... Finally someone said, 'right, shall we make a move?' And everyone started shuffling around getting ready to leave. Some of them took their time and others left quite quickly. It was their decision to go but I had edged them on.

Being a dinner party host is similar to being a uterus towards the end of pregnancy. Your uterus does everything it can to bring your baby into the world but it's a team effort. Your baby works with you. Some babies take longer to get ready and others move more quickly. Your uterus wants your baby to leave, it has prepared for this and it will do as much as possible to encourage your baby to be born. Try to be patient with your body.

YOUR PELVIS IN ACTION

Your pelvis is also shaping, moving and adapting for birth. Your ligaments and pelvis have both been heavily manipulated by a cocktail of hormones to allow as much room as possible for your baby. Your pubic joint can open by around a centimetre during labour. If you've ever slept in a king-sized bed after being in a double, you'll know how much difference that little bit of extra room makes! When it comes to making good use of this space, imagine you need to get a ring off your finger – you wouldn't pull it straight up and off would you? You would be twisting it at different angles to help it slide off. What you're doing with your ring there is similar to what you can do to help your baby come through your pelvis. Some women naturally start moving and rolling their hips or slightly squatting, so if you feel the need to move in a certain way, go with your body.

Towards the end of labour, there are ways to help keep your pelvis as open as possible and to help your baby into the ideal position. Aim to keep your knees as far away from your spine as possible as often as you can. For example, when you stand upright your knees are as far away from your pelvis as they can be. When you sit try to have your knees lower than your pelvis.

KEY POINTS

- Trust the relationship your body has with your baby: your uterus wants to get your baby out.
- Your baby's head changes shape to fit through your pelvis.
- Help your baby into the ideal position by being aware of your posture and movement during pregnancy.

Birth for your baby

WHEN WE THINK and talk about labour, we almost always focus on women being in labour and forget that babies experience labour too. As you know, their head can change shape to adapt their position and they very much do their bit to come into the world as easily as possible. As none of us remember being born, it is hard to know how babies feel. There are several theories about the impact of birth on babies and their feelings after birth, but the fact is, no one really knows for sure. What we do know is that babies are conscious, aware, and are very much experiencing labour too. Here we will run through birth through the eyes of a newborn, so that you can understand how to help to create the best possible environment for your baby to be born into.

A SPA DAY

Imagine you've been given a free spa day and you're chilling in the jacuzzi, where it is lovely and warm. The sounds you can hear are consistent and the volume is generally at the same level. People are coming in and out, but no one is bothering you because you're in your own little bubble and the noise of the jacuzzi is making voices more muffled. The lighting is dim. You've got food and drink whenever you want it and you don't really need anything else. It's a predictable environment and you're pretty settled. After a while, you know it's time for you to leave.

To leave the jacuzzi you need to go through a tight tunnel, and you don't know where the tunnel is going to lead to. Suddenly the water around you drains and a strong force is pushing you into the tunnel and out of the jacuzzi. You do your best to go along with it but you still have no idea where you're going to come out.

The force gets stronger and stronger, everything is getting a bit squashed, and you become very aware of each part of your body as the tunnel gets smaller and smaller. You have to twist and turn your body to fit through. You're okay but your head is beginning to get squashed. At one point you wonder if you are stuck but then the tunnel clears, giving you a bit more room. This extra room means you can wriggle around to get through. The sensation of being squeezed and pushed gets pretty intense. You're wondering, is this definitely the way to the exit? Where am I going to come out?

Your friends are waiting outside to meet you and they've been waiting for a while so they are really excited. They have lots of towels to dry you with, a new camera with a bright flash, your favourite food ready they are very EXCITED about seeing you.

You go through one final squeeze and ... whoa, you're out. There's so much space it's scary. Your arms fly wide open; you had no idea your arms could open that wide. Someone grabs you, rubs you with a towel, puts a hat on you, everything is so loud and it seems so bright! The high-pitched noises, the cooler temperature, the brightness, it's all a bit much and your body needs to adjust to all of these changes. As your eyes are starting to adjust, a very bright flash goes off in your face and disorientates you. All the sensory stimulation is overwhelming. Then lastly, someone shoves food in your mouth. How would you feel?

A baby is born into an entirely new universe. They have never seen light, heard clear sounds, been touched, and most importantly, been independent from you. It is difficult to explain how sensitive a newborn baby is. The jacuzzi and tunnel are the nearest I could come up with and just one way of explaining how overwhelming a massive change of environment can be. There's a lot more that a baby experiences at birth – they now have some responsibility for themselves too, even if they're not conscious of it; their bodies start to do things immediately that they have never done before. Their circulation switches over (so oxygenated blood starts to run through the arteries, and deoxygenated blood now runs through the veins), they need to breathe, regulate their own body temperature and feed. Life as they knew it has completely changed.

Going from floating around being kept warm and fed through your belly button to being pushed and squeezed out into the world must be a strange experience. However, it's really important to know that being squeezed is not a bad thing, so please don't think that you want to prevent this for your baby. The squeezing helps to loosen and release the mucus and fluid in their lungs and airways so they can breathe easier. Not only that, your body has prepared vaginal flora (bacteria) for your baby to kick start their immune system. This particular flora is symbiotic with your breastmilk, meaning that your baby's gut will have the perfect bacteria to digest your milk. Your body is so in sync with your baby.

HOW TO HELP YOUR BABY ADJUST TO THEIR NEW WORLD

Dim lighting and quiet voices are good for you in labour, as we have covered (see page 168), and they are good for a baby coming into the world too. To help your baby feel safe and calm your baby needs to be kept as close as possible to life as they knew it. The first main sources of comfort outside the womb are your:

- smell
- touch
- sound and your voice

Newborns will recognise and trust their mum's smell, touch and voice.

Smell
In all animals, including humans, smell is the oldest of the five senses and plays a huge role in many behaviours that are essential for survival and reproduction. All mammals react to odours and your newborn baby is no different. A newborn baby's incredible sense of smell will never be as good in adult life. Unwashed newborns use their sense of smell as a comfort

measure by bringing their hands to their nose and mouth for that familiar smell. Research shows that babies will choose their mum's milk over anyone else's almost every time. In one study, when two different types of milk were placed either side of a baby's head, they kept turning to the side that smells like their mum.

Skin-to-skin contact is so important after birth for sense of smell. If your baby needs to go to special care or is born prematurely, skin-to-skin contact is usually possible at some point. If it is not immediately possible, don't worry as it is still just as important even if this is a few days later. What you can do in this situation is to put something with your smell in their cot or incubator; the neonatal staff will be able to help guide you on what's safest. This simple thing brings back some familiarity for them. I recently watched an online clip where a dad puts a mum's T-shirt next to their newborn baby, and within seconds he stops crying. That is how powerful and important you and your body are to your baby.

The importance of touch

As well as being a comfort, touch is crucial for newborns. Touch through skin-to-skin contact, massage, or stroking, is known to improve weight gain, reduce stress, stabilise the respiratory system, prevent low blood sugar and reduce crying. Research shows that when premature babies are massaged daily, they gain weight faster and perform better in recognition tests. You know when you're feeling a bit vulnerable or down and someone close to you gives you a hug, it's like they have taken some of your burden away and you get a sense of relief. Babies get that too. In fact, for most of us, touch remains an important factor in our lives.

Skin-to-skin contact after birth is so important and your midwife will help you bring your baby to your chest as soon after birth as possible. This is simply where you have your naked baby placed on your chest, touching just your skin; it does what it says on the tin, skin-to-skin. Leaving them in skin-to-skin for at least one hour after birth really helps to gently introduce them into their new world. Without any skin-to-skin contact it can be hard for a newborn to feel safe on their own. Not only that, they are kept nice and warm and warm babies feed better. Keeping them warm also helps to stabilise blood sugars because they do not need to spend precious energy on regulating their own temperature; you're helping them to do that so they remain an extension of your body. If you are unable to have skin-to-skin, for whatever reason, get your birth partner to do it instead; your baby will still get many of the benefits feeling soothed and comforted and it is a great bonding experience for them too.

If you leave your baby in skin-to-skin contact on your chest your baby will naturally start to head towards food when they are ready. There are some fascinating videos of this happening on YouTube, one in particular called 'breast crawl' with over a million views. So after trying for a while (apparently it was almost 45 minutes in total) at 7 minutes 30 seconds the baby latches himself onto the breast – with no guidance. This isn't always possible but it goes to show just how instinctive newborn behaviour is.

Sometimes we can be a bit impatient about breastfeeding and want a baby to feed right away after birth, but if we go back to how you felt when you had just come out of the 'jacuzzi' on your spa day, all of the surrounding distractions meant that you were not initially interested in food. Rather than have food put in your mouth, you would probably want it left in reach ready for when you had adjusted and felt hungry. That is what staying in skin-to-skin gives your baby the opportunity to do – get the food when they feel ready. They may start to show you that they are ready to eat by turning their head, licking their lips and sucking their hands; if you want to encourage them and bring them onto the breast, that's up to you. The important part is waiting for them to be ready, if you can.

Familiar sounds

The sound of your heartbeat and voice are the most familiar sounds your newborn knows. Having your baby in skin-to-skin on your chest brings them closer to your heart and voice, and therefore the familiar comfort of the womb. You don't have to do anything, just hearing you talk is enough.

Your partner's voice and those that you have spent a lot of time with after 24 weeks in pregnancy will also be familiar to your baby. If you can't have skin-to-skin at birth, your birth partner should be able to do this instead, and their voice will be comforting too.

KEY POINTS

- Your baby is also experiencing labour.
- Your body and baby are so in sync.
- Your baby does not yet understand their new world and outside stimuli can be overwhelming.
- Newborns need your body in order to feel safe.
- The first main sources of comfort outside the womb are your smell, touch and sound.

When a baby is born, so is a mother

THIS SECTION IS one of the shortest of the book but it has an important message. Healthcare professionals rarely tell women about the 'birth pause' and rarely do mums know or talk about it amongst themselves. Some mums even tell me that they are embarrassed or feel guilty about how they felt in the first few moments after birth, when there's no need to be. So let's talk about it now.

The raw emotion that pours out in this life-changing moment is incredible and can be overwhelming. The moment you meet the one you have been nurturing and carrying for months whilst flooded with hormones, determination and vast physiological changes, cannot be put into words. You will only ever experience birth a select number of times, which is why you need to know about the birth pause.

In a world where everything moves so quickly, we need to make a specific effort to pause and absorb what has just happened – you did it! Whatever way you gave birth, you did it. You're a mother.

Most women become still during the moments just after their baby's arrival, no matter what type of birth they have had. There's a 'birth pause' where the world seems to stop, when those first few moments are surreal. Some new mums have told me that they feel guilty because they didn't want to hold their baby right away. I've seen women almost 'guard' themselves and lean back when I have gone to pass them their baby immediately. Over the years I have come to appreciate that it is completely normal not to hold your baby instantly.

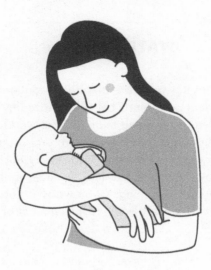

Just like in lots of other milestones that life has to offer, there is no one way to go into motherhood.

I once cared for a woman having a water birth, she was incredible; she was so calm and focused throughout her labour. When the baby was born she just looked down, staring at her baby under the water. I slowly helped bring her baby to the surface and let her just look and have a moment to come back into herself and be present. Nothing was needed from her in that moment; her mind and body had worked hard to get here and she took a pause. Me, dad and mum all looked at the baby with his little face sitting out of the water and cord still pulsating, delivering oxygen-rich blood to him. After about 20 seconds he screwed up his nose, opened his eyes and looked around before filling his lungs with air and taking his first breath. This all took less than a minute and I just had my hands gently supporting him to stay above the water until mum felt *ready* to bring him up to her chest in skin-to-skin. If she had given birth on the bed, floor or pretty much anywhere else I would not have touched her baby. I would have supported her to sit back and look at her baby in peace. It was only because the baby was under water that I helped him come to the surface to breathe and take that all-important breath.

WATER BIRTHS

Babies that are born in water can take a little longer to take their first breath and may seem particularly calm or unfazed by the whole thing. Water is a gentle way of bringing them into the world; they have gone from water to water, it is still nice and warm and usually the lights are dim. Your midwife may wait for your baby to cry but then may ask to stimulate your baby if they need a little reminder that they have been born and need to start breathing. Don't worry if this happens – your midwife knows what to do and when to intervene, if at all.

Afterwards she said that she will never forget that moment as she watched her son take his first breath so calmly. Like many women, this mum really needed a moment herself to appreciate what had happened to her and her body. She needed to pause and just look at her baby first.

Her first birth was very different because she didn't realise that the birth pause existed. She explained that before she knew it, her baby was on her chest and her arms felt 'weird and wobbly', so having to hold the baby wasn't the pleasurable experience she had expected. Her gut instinct made her want to get the baby off of her. She said that it was too overwhelming and told me that she felt bad for feeling like that for months afterwards and didn't understand why. But this was just a reaction, not a conscious thought or action.

It's quite common for mums to be a little stunned, physically drained or relieved at first; something changes permanently and it is a powerful moment. Almost always the first tears I see are from the partner or the birth partner. You have gone from a place of hard work and focus to suddenly stopping, relaxing your muscles and then seeing your baby for the first time. If you have been in 'the zone' your mammalian brain is still very active and it takes a moment to come back into the human thinking or neocortical way of thinking. Unless there has been a problem in labour or a concern over the wellbeing of your baby, there's no rush; relish the moment and enjoy the pause.

Overall, women have more peaceful, memorable and better birth experiences if we move away from having expectations about those first few moments. You might cry at first, or you might not. It is a time to be in this fleeting moment. It is a chance to take in the details; their tiny toes, fingers and face. If your baby is directly on your chest sometimes you can't see them properly. A short pause before skin-to-skin contact won't make any difference to a healthy baby and unless the baby needs a little more support from your midwife, we all have time to pause.

Unless told otherwise, midwives often assume women want us to pass them their baby right away and some women do want this. Put your preference in your birth plan so your midwife knows what you want and feels comfortable to stand back.

No matter what kind of birth you have, if it feels right, pause and breathe. If you want to pick your baby up right away and you don't feel the need for a pause then great. Just don't *expect* anything at all from yourself right away.

KEY POINTS

- The first few moments following birth are precious.
- You might not want to hold your baby right away, you may need to pause.
- No one should rush you unless there is a true emergency – you're the boss.
- Write about the pause in your birth plan so your midwife knows to hold off, if this is what you want.
- You're going to be a great mum.

Real birth stories

Amy's story

I was 41 weeks exactly and had a midwife appointment in the morning and took up the offer of a sweep. I went for it as I was so ready to meet our baby girl. I met the other antenatal girls afterwards who were also patiently waiting for babies to decide to arrive! We felt hot and fed up. Walking back I wondered if I was getting contractions. I had lots of Braxton Hicks the whole week so assumed not. By the time I was home at 2pm I was definitely having contractions. I gave it some time to make sure it wasn't a false alarm and called my husband to tell it was happening.

I took paracetamol and kept busy. As they got stronger I put my TENS machine on and went up on the levels as they progressed. Tried to keep occupied watching Netflix. I liked the premise and ideas of hypnobirthing so tried as much of the breathing techniques as I could and managed well as the contractions got to 2–3 minutes apart and pretty intense.

By 10pm I was ready to go to hospital. I was seen around 11pm and was 'almost 4cm'! I was offered pain relief and suggested to go home. My body was telling me no, I didn't want to leave. I didn't fancy the suggestion to, 'Have a walk round the car park' so asked for some pethidine and got a bit of rest while it worked its magic. James tried to get some rest too but was a bit wired with everything going on. At around 1am the contractions kicked up a notch and I woke up. I was 5cm and was walked (very slowly) up to a labour room. I'd had some bleeding so to keep an eye we went there with potential for a midwife-led pool room later on. I'd liked the idea of bobbing round in a birthing pool.

I got on the gas and air and was convinced it wasn't plugged in; the contractions felt like they were stacking up on each other. My TENS was constantly on boost! I was in the zone. In a good position leaning on the bed. Keeping my hips moving. James was great; when he heard my breathing getting erratic he would remind me to slow down.

The belt wasn't getting a good trace of baby's heartbeat as I was moving a lot. The midwife suggested using a clip on her head to get a more reliable reading. There was fun and games getting on the bed for this! Every time I lifted my leg a contraction started and I couldn't get up! Finally, just before 2.30am I was heaved on the bed. The clip was attached and, lo and behold, I was 10cm dilated! 'So I can push?' I asked. 'If you feel like it.' The midwife popped to go get supplies for the usual long, first-time mum pushing stage.

At 2.32 I felt the urge and went with it after holding back previously. It was totally instinctive, I'd moved onto my right side.

James looked down and saw the head appear! Luckily, just as he thought he might have to deliver his own daughter the midwife was back!

There was no stopping me.

Push 2 her head was out.

Push 3 and our daughter was born.

2.39am, 8.6.18.

12.5 hours start to finish.

I surrendered to the labour. It was tough but quick. I went with it. I felt like I was in a haze but the moment she was handed to me everything cleared. Our gorgeous healthy Ella was here.

Laura's story, first-time mum
At 27 I was lucky enough to become pregnant for the first time. As a registered nurse and a practising health visitor it was the opinion of many that pregnancy, labour and the care of a newborn baby would be a breeze for me as I 'knew what I was doing'. My pregnancy was pretty much uncomplicated until around

32 weeks pregnant when my blood results were abnormal and I began the weekly journey to the hospital for blood tests and monitoring of baby due to possible cholestasis (a condition where bile cannot flow from the liver to the duodenum).

I saw two consultants, one who was happy to keep an eye on me and one who suggested an induction at 37 weeks. In the end I was brought in for induction of labour at 37+5, which lasted four long days, ending in an emergency Caesarean. Our beautiful baby girl Elsie was born weighing 7lbs 11ozs at 00.02am on the 11th December 2016.

Despite it being midnight, the team were great and they allowed us to remain in theatre for 45 minutes with skin-to-skin to initiate breastfeeding. I was really eager to try the breast crawl as a natural instinct, and mummies, it is an amazing natural instinct! So very clever!

I was exhausted, but due to the hospital's protocol of early mobilisation I was up eight hours later walking to the bathroom. (In hindsight, I realise this was necessary to prevent post-surgery complications.) I desperately wanted to breastfeed but was very tired; thankfully, an amazing midwife helped me to hand-express my colostrum and sat with me for over two hours, which I will forever be grateful for! On day two we were discharged home.

The following four months were very tough. I struggled to sleep between feeds due to flashbacks of a traumatic birth and I wished the days and nights by. I smiled on the forefront and put on a brave face. Due to C-section recovery breastfeeding was tough to establish. As sleep deprivation took its toll I hit rock bottom. I felt I had lost all sense of who I was and as though I was just going through the motions of each day. With encouragement from my family I sought help from a GP who signposted me to the IAPT (improving access to psychological therapies) team and the health visitors, and prescribed me medication for PTSD (post-traumatic stress disorder) and postnatal depression.

Depression in the postnatal period can happen to anybody. It does not stereotype.

I wanted to share my experience to show that it does not matter who you are, what job you do, or which culture you come from, when you are given a newborn baby you are a mother and we are all together in the same boat. Those months were hard and I had to dig deep but now feel lucky that the experience has made me who I am today a strong woman and mother who has an unbreakable bond with her now two-year-old little girl.

I went back to work over 18 months ago as a health visitor and was initially very nervous. However, I feel my experiences with PTSD and PND have given me a level of empathy I did not have before, and as such I am a huge advocate for promoting mental health services and talking about our feelings.

My birth experience was far from ideal, but there are lots of services out there: midwives, health visitors, GPs, perinatal mental health teams, IAPT, to name a few. I am eternally grateful for the professionals who supported me and am now able to say that two years on the experience has not put me off trying for another baby in the future, and my partner of nine years and I get married next year.

Jordan, second-time mum
I fell pregnant with baby number two when my first born was 13 months old. My first pregnancy ran so smoothly and I had a lovely home water birth and naturally wanted the same with my second.

At my booking appointment my midwife was super-supportive and encouraging of my decision to have a home birth. After the usual checks they do, I received a letter in the post to say I needed to see a consultant and have two extra growth scans due to having low PAPP-A (pregnancy associated plasma protein A). I still don't really know what it is but it's something about the placenta – which can affect the baby's growth. There was mentions of risk of Down's syndrome, still birth and miscarriages, which shocked me completely and turned my positive pregnancy into one of anxiety.

I went for my first growth scan at 30 weeks and all was well. The consultant, however, insisted I had a hospital birth and I kept saying no. She bartered down to a birth-centre birth but you are the same risk level as home birth then, so what was the difference? My midwife kept reassuring me I would be ok for a home birth.

The next growth scan at 35 weeks again showed that my baby was growing fine. I thought they would discharge me back under the community team and I could continue down my positive home birth route. But this time I saw a different consultant who suggested an extra third growth scan and said due to my BMI being high (it's one point over to warrant me being overweight) that it wouldn't be safe for me to have a home birth. I felt at a loss: it was me vs them, and they're the experts in the field with the fancy letters after their names. I get it – they need to cover their backs if anything goes wrong but surely the buck should stop with me?

I went for my third growth scan at 38 weeks and the measurements looked great so I was feeling so positive that I would finally be discharged. But once again they said no. This time the consultant reeled off a load of worrying statistics in relation to my BMI that I'd be X times more likely to need an instrumental birth or C-section and that I was even too high risk for the birth centre. He even told me he'd want me to be induced ASAP. It angered me so much I cried angry tears and kept asking why, and to justify his reasons. He blamed the BMI and said he has to treat everyone whose BMI is high whether they're 35 or 75, and that's a big difference. In short, I told him I am having a home birth and walked out the hospital feeling like I could conquer the world.

I told myself I AM going to have the birth I planned even if I ended up in hospital. I wasn't going to give in or let their worry of getting a disciplinary get in the way of one of the most amazing experiences a woman can have.

Less than two weeks later I went into labour spontaneously at home. I was in my birth pool listening to some chilled music whilst my best friend, who is a student midwife, poured water over my back and my husband kept me hydrated. Three hours later out came my beautiful daughter; I just felt relief that nothing had gone wrong and that my stubbornness and intuition had paid off.

I didn't do anything specifically to help me relax like hypnobirthing or music etc. It was really down to the reassurance of my midwife. It also helped that the same midwife, Emma, that I saw throughout my pregnancy came to me in labour. I didn't have that experience first time around because I lived in a different area and they had a designated home-birth team, whereas this time round, the community and home-birth team are the same and cover the same area.

During the labour I did get into my 'zone', but I didn't prepare for that, I just did it.

Hannah's story
@the_savvy_mummy

We found out whilst away for the weekend that I was pregnant (for the fifth time) after realising that I was super-emotional and hormonal. I was so nervous after we had been trying for a couple of years.

After my first baby I had three miscarriages, one which was really horrid and ended in a blood transfusion. We wanted to wait until we had the three-month okay before I started to believe it and tell anyone.

Everything looked normal at 12 weeks but it took a lot of hypnobirthing and meditation for me to get in the right headspace throughout pregnancy.

We had extra scans the whole way through the pregnancy, which really made me feel reassured and that if anything was to look or feel suspicious we would find out straight away.

My pregnancy was fab the whole way through; it did seem tougher this time around as I was a lot more tired. I also had SPD, which is quite painful, so I went for regular massages and did lots of exercises, which kept it at bay.

I learned not to focus on my due date too much but the pregnancy flew by and all of a sudden I was 10 days overdue! The midwife recommended I book in for an induction and sweep. I declined these as I believed in my body and I knew baby would arrive when baby was ready. I even went to my best friends' wedding three days before I gave birth!

Hypnobirthing was incredible and I would recommend it to everyone. I kept a space mask on for most of the labour to block out the rest of the world, when I transferred from my house to the hospital I even had a blanket over my head! I listened to a hypnobirthing app non-stop and totally got in a Zen zone.

The midwives didn't believe, when I arrived at the hospital, that I was anywhere near the end as I was so calm.

I let them check me and I was 6cm dilated so they ran the pool and I got in; this was such a great relief, the pool was lovely.

After about two hours I told them I could feel the baby coming, I was so calm I don't think they believed me.

My baby was born in the water so easily and calmly. The midwives were a little shocked because I was so calm. I managed to get my sister to film the birth on her phone for me as after all the hypnobirthing practice I really wanted to see it for myself. It was truly beautiful and makes me want to have more!

Juno was born at 6.45am on 10.10.19 in the most magical water birth I could ever have wished for.

I was the first one in the world to touch her and I brought my baby up from the water into the word and hubby cut the cord. We had skin-to-skin straight away and Juno latched on as soon as I tried to breastfeed. She has fed well ever since.

Giving birth like this taught me so much about my mind and body. I gained a sense of understanding and strength I never knew I had. After all the pregnancies that didn't work out I honestly felt something would go wrong my whole pregnancy. It was only when I really got into hypnobirthing and meditating that I started to relax and trust my body.

If I could have that labour again I would do it tomorrow!

Heidi's story
@heidijanetransk

On 14th September 2018, I discovered I was pregnant again, eight months post C-section. My initial thoughts were excitement again, and then fear. Fear of how safe this pregnancy would be and fear of another C-section where I felt numb.

I didn't want to feel any of that. So I looked into hypnobirthing, which came from a comment from a mum I met in my community who taught hypnobirthing and mentioned it to me. I replied with 'ah I had a C-section so I don't think it would help me?' HOW WRONG WAS I!

Hypnobirthing is for *every* birth and changed my outlook on the impending delivery. For me, it was the wording and affirmations, teaching your brain to trust your body, and the path of birth for that body and baby. To put in context, words like 'contractions' become 'surges' and my language surrounding Peggy's birth was noticeably more positive.

I was seen by my midwife and never once was a repeat belly birth forced on me. It was so reassuring to feel I had a choice! I planned for a VBAC (vaginal birth after C-section) and felt supported and informed by the healthcare professionals looking after me.

For myself, I consented to continuous fetal monitoring (as it made me feel more relaxed) during labour, and it felt right for us.

At 20 weeks, we discovered our baby had suspected renal pelvic dilatation and would need to have repeat scans at 28 weeks and 36 weeks. Our plans for VBAC remained unaffected, following advice from our consultants that our baby was well.

In preparation, I also had researched 'gentle C-sections' and how many of the 'natural' birth elements can be applied (where safe) to belly births, in case this situation arose again.

I approached birth with excitement and when my due date came and went, I didn't feel frustrated and just enjoyed the last few days of being pregnant (you truly miss that bump!).

At my 40-week appointment (two days after my due date) my midwife measured my bump and I was measuring small for dates. Having had a larger baby before I thought this was a bit odd! It was also the third time I had measured small and so we were sent in for a heart trace and potential scan to make sure baby was well.

I was advised to be induced going post-dates. However, I was given a few more days to see if things would happen on their own (I was already 1cm dilated) as baby was moving okay.

This decision to agree to induction came from an affirmation I had been taught: 'I make informed decisions that feel right for me and my baby'. With her issues with her kidneys, I couldn't risk she might have been unwell.

That date came and off we went to be induced. I was for trial of a Cook Cervical Ripening Balloon Catheter, but when they examined me I was already 3cm! So my waters were released instead, it was 4pm. ...

The labour ward was packed and so I stayed on the antenatal ward, but my surges were coming quick and fast! However, I zoned out, kept the lighting low (it helped that it was evening) and listened to my affirmations; I couldn't even hear the other women.

At 10pm I was moved to the labour ward and again created our birth space in the room. We had soft music, I took Wilfred's bobble hat as an anchor and I felt totally relaxed (despite very intense surges).

Another four hours and little progress. It was the first time I felt scared and frustrated, but I had learnt not to let that emotion in, and thought logically to get an epidural and at least rest until my next exam and conserve some energy.

Despite this logical thinking, my epidural only worked on one side so I was battling surges for a couple of hours before I moved on my side (by advice of my lovely midwife) and it took effect at last!

Another exam, still 5cm. Again frustration crept in. Our obstetrician suggested we try a drip ... and I initially agreed.

Then I heard: 'I am preparing for the birth of a calm baby and a confident mother' and I decided my body had done enough, and I didn't want an emergency situation. I also was informed that risk of rupture could increase with the drip.

I burst into tears, and the release gave me the strength to know our baby needed to be born by belly, so she was calm and safe.

At 7.46am Peggy arrived weighing 8lbs. She was placed onto my chest and we had immediate skin-to-skin and she fed about 20 minutes after her birth.

It wasn't uncomplicated, and I suffered a post-partum haemorrhage on the operating table, but knew I was in the safest hands.

In recovery, our OB who delivered her came to see us and reassured us about what had caused the blood loss. He said it could have been scar tissue (from the previous section) or that I was on the border of rupturing.

I was so proud I had listened to my body and my baby at the time I did, and not had the drip.

I don't like the phrase 'unsuccessful' and so I won't say my VBAC was that. Unsuccessful would be if I didn't feel in control, which I did.

Despite a really heavy blood loss and abdominal delivery, Peggy breastfed well and actually lost no weight at her day-five check (when babies can lose up to 10 per cent), in fact she gained an ounce! 'My breast milk is just right for my baby.'

I want every woman preparing for a VBAC or a repeat C-section to know there is no 'failure'; your body is amazing, and birth can be beautiful, even when the unexpected arises.

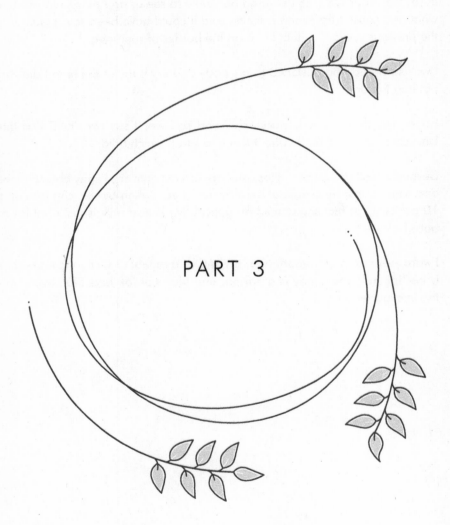

PART 3

Becoming Mum

~~~

Welcome to the world of new motherhood! This part of the book is all about the days after the birth and what to do after waving goodbye to your midwife.

We are going to run through what to expect, physically and mentally, how to look after your postpartum self, healing, breastfeeding and the most important things your newborn needs. There is also a helpful list of resources at the end. You can always call specific numbers for more individualised questions or help if you need it.

Your baby has now joined you inside your sacred circle (see page 5) and caring for both of you is going to be wonderfully exhausting. But the most important thing to remember now is that you are going to be an *amazing* mum.

WHAT I WOULD HAVE TOLD MY POSTPARTUM SELF

I was recently sent this message on social media and thought it was such good advice I had to share it with you (with permission, of course):

'After seeing so many amazing birthing stories, it has made me really think recently about what I would have told myself just [after my baby was born] and I was officially a MUM.

'I would have told myself to cut myself some slack. It's okay to cry sometimes (well, most of the time – I cried every time an advert with a baby came on the TV for months.) You're bloody emotional; your body has just gone through the biggest job of its life!

'Be realistic … leave your hair in a scruffy bun for as long as you need to and stay in your pyjamas as long as physically possible. I am the worst for putting myself under pressure to get up and get dressed. Accepting you have just brought a little human being into the world is the best thing you can do. It doesn't matter what you look like; you are Wonder Woman!

'I would have told myself to stay at home longer and not to try and do a big shop three days after having a Caesarean. Accept help from others: you can't do everything and you need rest. Big time!

'I would have told myself to sleep when the baby sleeps (sounds clichéd, I know) but I never did this, and wish I did. Everybody said this to me but I never listened. I always thought there were things that needed doing when Jett was asleep and then I was ratty by 2pm. This point could save your sanity; I lost mine trying to do it all.

'I would have told myself to do what is right for you and your baby and not judge yourself based on somebody else's opinion or experience. I was desperate to have a home birth and I was distraught when Jett arrived by C-section. I felt I had failed, even though this was out of my control. Things don't always go to plan but if you and baby are well, you are doing amazing.

'Lastly, I would tell myself to just enjoy the journey because every day is so precious. The washing can wait, the cleaning can wait, or you can order a takeaway. Somebody told me this before I had Jett and it is so true. Be patient, be emotional but mostly be present.'

The first 24 hours

THE FIRST 24 hours after birth are different for all women but at some point during this time you will say goodbye to the midwife who looked after you during labour and birth. If you're in a hospital or midwife-led unit (MLU) then it will be you that is going home, but if you had a home birth it will be your midwife heading off home or back to the office. Being without a midwife may feel daunting and it's the one thing that most new mums have in common. New mums often have a realisation that they don't know what comes next or what will happen from now on. So in this section we will run through your options after birth and what to expect.

THE GOLDEN HOUR

Let's look at the first hour after birth. Midwives no longer rush in to weigh the baby immediately – they are generally very protective over 'the golden hour', which is the first hour of your baby's life. That hour should be as undisturbed as possible as you both need time and space to appreciate what just happened. I mean, it doesn't get much bigger than giving life!

Ideally, you want to be in skin-to-skin contact with your baby for at least one hour after birth. Studies revealed that babies who were in skin-to-skin within two hours of birth had warmer feet 23 hours after birth. It was thought that this wasn't just because of the transfer of heat but because being in skin-to-skin with their mum reduced some of the stress of birth. Stress tends to divert blood from the extremities (like the feet) making them feel colder and cause more energy reserves to be used up. Which is possibly also why babies who have skin-to-skin soon after birth are better able to maintain their blood sugar levels. Skin-to-skin is one of the best gifts you can give your baby and it also has a huge impact on breastfeeding initiation (also see page 288). Midwives and birth experts have known for years that skin-to-skin and breastfeeding reduces the risk of bleeding after birth and increases natural oxytocin, but thanks to new research we now have a fancy name for this physiological process – 'pronurturance'.

If you have your baby in hospital you will stay in the birth room for at least an hour after birth, and usually for a couple of hours. NICE Guidelines also support this 'golden hour', unless there is a medical reason to separate or disturb you and your baby.

You may stay in skin-to-skin for longer but when you are ready your midwife will offer to give your baby vitamin K and to weigh your baby. Finding out the weight of your baby is a really exciting moment and answers the question everyone will ask. We make a note of the weight so we can check how baby is growing going forward. Then it is up to you what happens next – your baby can go back to you for more skin-to-skin or you can have a shower (or a bed bath if you've had a C-section), change of clothes and something to eat if you haven't already. Most women are really hungry after birth.

In the first few hours after birth your midwife will:

- Make sure you are generally feeling okay and do your observations (blood pressure, pulse, temperature, oxygen saturations and respiratory rate).
- Check your bleeding and perineum and give you pain relief if you need it.
- Weigh and check your baby over for anything physical like skin tags, etc.
- Help with feeding your baby, check your position and attachment, if needed.
- Answer any questions you may have and give reassurance.
- Get you some good old tea and toast.

Your midwife will be there just for you and will be able to help you with anything you need in those first couple of hours after birth. She will stay with you longer if you need more support though and carry out any further investigations that are needed.

THE NEXT FEW HOURS AND GOING HOME

If you have had a home birth and do not need to go into hospital for any reason, your midwife will make sure you are happy with everything, make sure you have all the contact details you need, good support from those around you, and will let you know when he/she or a colleague will next come to see you. Sometimes you will be offered a clinic appointment for your postnatal follow-up and your midwife can organise this with you before they leave.

If you have had your baby in a Midwife-led Unit (MLU) or hospital setting they'll ask you where you want to go, whether home or the postnatal ward. Generally, women that have had a vaginal birth with no complications can go home that same day – sometimes after a matter of hours. Other times women will go to the postnatal ward if they need a little more clinical care, such as observations or monitoring, but also if they'd like extra support with feeding overnight. If you have had a C-section then you will need to stay for at least one night. In some hospital units partners can stay and in others they can't (due to space or safety considerations). It is worth finding this out beforehand so that it isn't a shock if your partner needs to go home.

THE NIPE CHECK

The Newborn and Infant Physical Examination (or NIPE as we shorten it to), is a check that is recommended for all newborn babies and should be done within 72 hours of birth. It's a full MOT for newborns, a more in-depth check than the initial one your midwife did at birth. We tend to start at the head and work our way all the way down to their tiny toes. Whilst working our way down we check things like their eyes, the rate and the specific sound of the heart, their reflexes, genitalia and much more. Some midwives and most paediatricians do NIPEs but if you are at home or no one is able to when you have your baby, you'll be offered a follow-up appointment so your baby can have this check done.

When it is time to go home from the maternity unit or hospital (massive moment, yippee!) your midwife will give you a pack and explain a few key things; this pack has a lot of useful and important information in it and a lot of contact numbers. You probably won't take in all of the information right away, but remember to take a look at it when you can or get your birth partner to go through it all when you get home. The contact details will include how to get in touch with your community midwife, during usual working hours, or out of hours you can call the maternity triage line (usually the same number you call if you had questions in pregnancy). If you have any questions, worries or concerns, don't be afraid to give them a shout. Things like feeding, sleeping, taking care of your postnatal healing and any wounds, will probably come up that you aren't sure about, especially with your first. No question is a silly question.

You may also be given a red book which contains a record of your baby's growth, development and immunisations from 0–4 years (the long-term plan is to go digital with this, so you may be given online access instead of a physical copy).

YOUR TOP-TO-TOE CHECK-UP

Your midwife will usually come to see you at home or offer you a clinic appointment within the first 24–48 hours after birth. This varies around the country, but either way, you should hopefully see a midwife you have seen at some point during pregnancy. Just like you were offered during the antenatal period you will be offered the standard routine care plus extra appointments or involvement with professionals should you need it.

These postnatal checks are to make sure that you and your baby are well, so please feel free to talk openly to your midwife about how you are feeling and what's going on. We will never judge you; we don't care if there is a pile of dirty dishes in the sink, and we don't expect to be waited on. We aren't guests; we are simply there to help and support you.

Typically, at the 'top-to-toe' assessment we want to find out:

- If your blood pressure and general observations are normal for you.
- How you are feeling in yourself. You may be quite tired and tearful at times; that is very normal and we will talk about that more on page 313.
- How your breasts are feeling and whether you are breastfeeding or not. We will check to make sure you are comfortable and there is no sign of infection in your breasts (mastitis).
- What is happening with your tummy. You may get period-like 'after' pains – it's normal as your uterus contracts and shrinks back down to its normal size, most commonly when you breastfeed your baby.
- Your blood loss. Blood loss is known as 'lochia' and will probably seem like a heavy period in the first three days but it should settle and start to change colour to a brown, watery loss after around five days, but sometimes this change can take longer. We will also ask about any clots or smelly loss.
- How any wounds are, e.g. a C-section or perineal wound.
- If you are weeing and pooing okay. Going for a wee can feel weird in the first few days and you may not feel when you need to go (see page 247).
- How your legs and calves are. We will checking for red, hot, painful or swollen areas or if you are breathless even when resting, as these could be signs of a blood clot. You may be given a blood thinner after birth if you have had a C-section or if you are at an increased risk of blood clot (thrombosis).

WHAT TO EXPECT AFTER THE BIRTH

Your body needs time to recover and heal after the birth and there is a lot going on. Here are some of the things you might experience in the days and early weeks after the birth. Many postnatal women are concerned about bleeding and going to the toilet after birth. No matter how you give birth, vaginally or via C-section, you will bleed after birth, so let's look at that first.

Bleeding

Your body needs to lose the lining of the womb that your baby has nestled in for the past nine months. You will need to change your pads regularly, especially in the first two or three days after birth. You may get strong 'after pains' with the bleeding, especially while you are breastfeeding, and taking regular painkillers helps with this. Sometimes women loose clots after birth, and small or stringy clots are usually normal. If any clots are larger or look more like tissue you need to call your midwife/triage line to let someone know. What we are thinking about here is that maybe the whole of the placenta didn't come away at birth, meaning that there is possibly a bit still in your uterus. It might be hard for you to tell what it is that you are losing, but don't worry, that's not your job. If you are unsure call anyway, and as strange as this may sound ... save the blood clot or sanitary towel for us to look at. We are happy to look at anything to check if it is normal. I much prefer it when women save their worries for me because it is much easier to diagnose things or reassure them that it's normal.

Weeing

Sometimes your bladder just needs a little bit of retraining to remember what it needs to do following a birth. If you have had a C-section or an epidural you will have had a catheter fitted, and your bladder wouldn't have been filling and emptying like it normally does. It may feel a bit weird or swollen around your urethra (wee hole). In the very early days it can be normal not to feel when you need to go or leak a bit of urine en-route to the loo.

If you had a vaginal birth weeing can feel really weird and almost like your body doesn't belong to you. You may still not feel like you need to go to the loo, even when your bladder is full. To help remind your bladder, you may want to set an alarm every few hours to go for a wee. During the night, turn your alarm off and try to wee every time you feed your baby.

Drinking plenty of water and staying well hydrated is vital for the postnatal period; it reduces the risk of blood clots, helps restore your body after losing blood and prevents constipation. This will mean that you do need to wee, even if you don't feel like it. By setting an alarm you are helping your bladder to get full and empty, and repeat the process. This is simple and easy re-training.

After the first few days and with a bit of training, any leaking and weird sensations should start to go, but if it doesn't you need to tell your midwife as we can refer you and make sure you get extra support early on. If you get any pain, stinging or burning passing urine you need to let your midwife know as soon as possible as it could be an infection.

Things to look out for

When you are home or without a midwife around there are some important symptoms you need to look out for. The most concerning problems after birth are bleeding, infection, pre-eclampsia or blood clots in the legs and/or lungs. If you get any of the symptoms below you need to let your midwife know immediately. They are all treatable but letting us know immediately means that the conditions won't progress and we can manage them better.

Signs and symptoms	Possible condition
Sudden and profuse blood loss or persistent increased blood loss Faintness, dizziness or palpitations/tachycardia (faster than normal heart rate)	Postpartum haemorrhage
Fever, shivering, abdominal pain and/or offensive vaginal loss	Infection
Headaches accompanied by one or more of nausea, vomiting and/or visual disturbances (flashing lights) within the first 72 hours after birth	Pre-eclampsia/eclampsia
Calf pain, redness or swelling Shortness of breath or chest pain	Thromboembolism (blood clot)

KEY POINTS

- The first hour after birth should be as undisturbed and restful as possible.
- You will be able to go home after a few hours if everything is well.
- There are specific symptoms to look out for after pregnancy (see page 248) – early recognition means easier treatment.
- You will be given a lot of support and help and this continues after the birth.

Your physical recovery and wellbeing

THE EXPECTATION VS reality memes are blowing up on social media; some of them are brilliant and hilariously spot on. Jokes aside though, unrealistic expectations of life after birth can sometimes damage your confidence and body image. Unless you know a lot of women who have had babies, your expectation vs reality might be slightly skewed. This section is all about realigning this.

THE MYTH OF 'BOUNCING BACK'

There is no such thing as 'bouncing' back. No matter how a mum that has 'bounced' back appears to be on the outside or how flat her tummy is, she is still very much in a recovery process, physically and mentally. Recovery is never just skin-deep for postnatal women – it goes much, much deeper.

It took nine months to grow your baby and it can take as long, if not longer, for your body to recover. If you saw the size of your placenta you will be able to picture the size of the wound inside your uterus. I don't ever want you to feel afraid of what your body is going through, or down about how you look, so it's important that you understand the recovery process fully so that you can feel confident and positive in your own skin.

Everything is rushed and fast in our lives now: fast food, emails, same-day deliveries, WhatsApp ... the list goes on. We expect our bodies to run at the same speed, but our bodies do not work like that. Our economy and culture have significantly evolved over the past few hundred years, but our bodies are hardly any different. Your body will recover in its own time and if you try to rush your recovery and do too much too soon, you might not heal properly and may end up with long-term problems or pain.

'All great achievements require time'

— DAVID J SCHWARTZ

You may expect your tummy to go down to its pre-baby size quite quickly, but it generally takes longer than you think. After birth, the uterus goes through a process called involution where it starts to shrink back to its pre-pregnant state. It has stretched right up to the top of your abdomen and now it needs to get right back down into your pelvis. Everyone is different but, on average, it takes around six weeks to involute. In addition, all the internal organs that have been displaced by your baby need to go back into their natural position. Some women say that their tummy doesn't ever appear to be the same after birth, and some women look no different – both are normal. The type of birth you had, and your general health and fitness before pregnancy, all have an impact on how quickly your body recovers.

FOLLOW-UP APPOINTMENTS

You aren't on your own in these early few weeks, even if it seems like that sometimes! Midwives and midwifery support workers (MSWs) are there to help you if you have problems with breastfeeding and anything else you need. If you need an extra visit or some more support just let your community team know so someone can come and see you or invite you to a clinic.

Usually your midwives will discharge you from their care around day 10 after birth, but are able to look after you, answer questions, or refer you back into the maternity unit up until 28 days after birth. Your midwife will help you follow up with anything you need to and won't discharge you if there are any concerns; she will make sure you are fit to be discharged from our care. You will be given a lot of local contact numbers for different things but we are always happy to help and you can always call us for advice on the triage line or ring the NHS helpline 111, if quicker. After us, your health visitor will take over and will be able to help with things like feeding, sleeping and monitoring your baby's developmental checks up until your baby goes to school. A local health visitor should make contact with you before your midwife discharges you; sometimes they will make contact with you in pregnancy. You may also need to see an obstetrician if you had any pregnancy or postnatal complications.

You will need to book a general check up with your GP at six weeks to check how you are healing and discuss contraception and this is an opportunity for you to ask questions.

Here's a quick run down from Dr Shireen, London GP and Instagrammer @doctorshireen:

'The "six-week check" is part of the NHS Newborn and Infant Physical Examination (NIPE) programme. The second NIPE check (your baby has the first one within 72 hours) is usually carried out by your GP and comprises of a physical examination of your baby and a review of their development. We often combine this with your postnatal check – although this may vary at different GP practices. This is an opportunity for us to offer some health promotion – this can include immunisations, breastfeeding/advice on weaning, car safety and dental health (although some of this may have already been covered by your health visitor). It also provides an opportunity for you to express any concerns you may have.

'During your postnatal check, we would have a general discussion about your mental health and wellbeing (and you will be screened for symptoms of postnatal depression).

'We also check your physical health – this involves a blood pressure check and if there are any concerns, an examination of your vulva to ensure your stitches have healed/are not infected (if you've had an episiotomy) or to take a swab if you've been having any unusual vaginal discharge. If you had a Caesarean section and have any concerns, we would check the scar for healing and to ensure there is no infection and perform an abdominal examination.

'Following this, we would have a chat about contraception methods (which differ in the postnatal period) and if you're overweight or obese, we can offer weight-loss advice and guidance in the postnatal period.

'Remember, this part of the postnatal check is about YOU – it's important to tell your doctor if you're struggling or feeling sad or anxious. These are all very common feelings in the postnatal period and there is so much support we can offer.

'Another common symptom that many women struggle with is incontinence – struggling to hold in their wee or sometimes poo. If that's the case for you, then again – please discuss this with your doctor, as there are so many possible treatment options.'

LOOKING AFTER YOURSELF

It is so important to look after yourself at this time; your baby needs you to feel as well as possible. There is one thing that speeds up recovery and works for everyone: nurturing yourself, resting, and setting boundaries for visitors. You need to take care of yourself so that you can be the best version of yourself, get better, and be able to care for your baby in the days, weeks and months ahead!

'Give it TIME. I just took it a week at a time, knowing each day would hurt a little less and I would be able to do more and feel better. I didn't put any pressure on myself to go out, I cancelled visitors when I needed to, and just sat with my baby. I felt selfish but only because I am a people-pleaser; for the first time in my life I also felt assertive and liberated by only doing what I wanted to do and I think that really helped. I always thought if anyone had a problem with it they weren't a good enough friend anyway.'

Katie, first-time mum

Healing your postnatal body and the importance of your recovery can easily be pushed aside as caring for your newborn takes over. Sometimes women will ignore their own discomfort or symptoms and just press on. Please try not to do this. Report any pain or anything you are unsure of and spend *at least* the first two weeks healing and recovering at home. No matter what type of birth you have had, you and your baby need to recover together. It may have been the perfect planned home water birth or it may have been a birth with a lot of intervention. Either way, you and your baby have been through one of the biggest physical and emotional transformations in life. It is very normal to ask your midwives lots of questions and it is totally acceptable to opt for rest over getting tasks done.

POSTNATAL PRACTICES AROUND THE GLOBE

~~~~~

Taking good care of yourself and focusing on your healing is not a luxury – it's an absolute necessity – and we haven't quite got to grips with that concept in the Western world. Below are some experiences about recovery and the postnatal period from around the world; we have a lot to learn from them.

In **Malaysia**, the postnatal period is considered to be six weeks after birth. During this time new mums are treated like queens. A new mother's sole focus is to rest and recover so she can build strength for motherhood. During the postnatal period there is a heavy emphasis on nurturing, nourishing and energising the new mother. Traditionally, those caring for postnatal women want them to be able to embrace motherhood, breastfeeding and the general demands that come with caring for a newborn.

In **China,** postpartum care is one of the most important traditions for women. Women will tend to stay home for the first month (known as the 'one-month sitting') and postnatal recovery is taken very seriously. The Chinese see it as an investment and once again ensure new mothers are well rested. The family take away demands and do as much as possible for the new mum. I was once told off by a Chinese grandmother for asking a woman to pull her own maternity knickers down so I could look at her C-section wound; she stopped me and said, 'Do not ask her to do anything, I do everything!' And that told me! Grandma insisted on doing everything and was very protective over her granddaughter's healing time.

As a side note: while there are definitely benefits to plenty of rest, the risk of blood clots might increase when women are totally bed-bound for one month, so a bit of moving about is probably a good thing!

In **The Netherlands,** all new mums get Kraamzorg (postnatal care at home). The Dutch believe postnatal recovery is a matter of national interest. This includes access to a maternity nurse who works in connection with mum, baby and their midwife/doctor. Usually the nurse provides 48 hours of care over 8–10 days and helps the new mum to care for herself physically and emotionally, as well as for her new baby. They also clean bathrooms, bedrooms and help with light household chores, so the mum can rest and recover.

Mexico has one of the largest and most diverse indigenous populations in Latin America and they speak around 62 languages in total. One thing the members of this diverse population all have in common is a great appreciation for postnatal recovery and focus on the first 40 days after birth. One thing that I find interesting is the use of plants from their region for herbal baths and teas. They also focus on warm nutritious foods to help heal and 'seal' the postnatal woman. The *cerrada de cadera*, translated as 'closing of the hips', is a gentle pressure bandage to help close the body of a mother. It is believed that in pregnancy and birth the mother needs to open and create, but now she needs to close and become a new woman, a mother. Postpartum sealing is practised soon after birth and continued through 40 days postpartum. This care is believed to restore mums quicker, enhance bonding and breastmilk production, prevent womb ailments and arthritis later on in life. Full-body massage is used to help heal and relax the mother.

In **India,** the practice of Ayurveda (a traditional mind–body health system) teaches that the first 40 days of life will affect the next 40 years of life. This is because the influence of the mother will naturally impact on her newborn so mum needs to regain her strength. Again there is a heavy focus on resting and eating warming foods that will help her return to balance; this includes foods that are easy to digest such as rice, and warming ingredients such as ginger, turmeric, pepper and herbs. Full-body massage is also included in postnatal care too as this helps circulation and promotes healing.

Many ancient and global traditions have a few things in common:

- New mum **rests** as much as possible.
- No expectation for mum to do it all – help is on hand.
- The first 40 days or four weeks is protected recovery time.
- Postnatal recovery = investment in long-term health for mum and baby.
- Eating warming and nourishing foods.

If the importance of postnatal recovery is known globally and has been highly regarded for hundreds perhaps thousands of years, then it is important for us to remember this. Many other things move a lot faster and we want things now, now, now, but rushing recovery doesn't do anything other than put further strain on the body.

'Our Western society has stolen this sacred time away from women because we think being back out with a hot #postbabybod is some kind of #goalz. Because on top of everything else, women should be expected to push out a baby and look fine five minutes later. We are not fine. We should not be expected to be fine. We are still bleeding. Our organs are still trying to find their way back home. Our babies need us to be focused on them entirely so we can regulate our hormones. And we need a lot of support from friends and family to do that. Because if, like most of the women in the Western world these days, we miss this vital window of bonding and healing and nurturing, it can have long-lasting [like, *years* ...] physical and mental health effects on the mother. I wish someone had told me how to care for my sister better. What food to bring her. What tea she needed. How to massage her. So if there is one thing I'd say to a mother of a newborn; stay in bed with your baby. You have nothing to prove. You are a fucking badass for sitting in your PJs, bonding with your newborn and accepting help. And if anyone thinks you're being dramatic or indulgent, throw this book at their head.'

Claire, mum of four, @jetsetmama

POSTNATAL WOUND CARE

Having some sort of wound in your vagina and perineum area is very common. About 350,000 women per year in the UK (that's up to 50 per cent) and millions more worldwide have perineal stitches. If you don't have any stitches or a tear you may have a C-section wound. Most wounds heal beautifully but to help you heal as quickly as possible, the key is to prevent infection. If you get an infection this will delay healing a bit and can be painful. The three key things are:

1. Any wound dressings may be changed by your midwife after 48 hours after your C-section, especially if there is any leaking from the wound. Avoid touching your dressing or wound.

2. Recommendations vary around the UK but any non-dissolvable stitches or beads will usually be taken out by your midwife after five to seven days, who will also advise you on how to further care for your wound depending on how it is healing.
3. Do not use any creams or soaps on your wound – just use warm water and pat dry with a clean towel daily.
4. Keep the general groin area clean and wear loose cotton clothing.
5. Use maternity pads because they are usually larger and smoother and don't pull on or irritate any stitches further. Change them often.
6. Wash your hands regularly, especially after you have changed your baby's nappy and of course every time you go to the loo yourself.

If you notice your wound is smelly, weeping or green/pussy, red, hot, swollen, you have more pain in the wound or your tummy than you had before, get unpleasant vaginal discharge or if you feel feverish and/or have a high temperature, you need to call your midwife as soon as possible – these are all signs of an infection.

Perineal wound

Your midwife may ask to have a look at your perineum to check for infection and make sure it is healing well. I always advise women to have a look themselves, as it can be very reassuring! This is not for everyone, so if you don't want to look at it, then don't force yourself. A lot of the women who do have a look say that it doesn't look as bad as they imagined or as bad as it feels. It is kind of like when you get a spot; it feels massive on your face but when you see it in the mirror it is nowhere near as bad. Having a look yourself is also good because you can monitor your own healing over the next few weeks so you will be able to see how well it is healing and detect any changes yourself.

HELP WITH HEALING

There is a lot you can do for yourself to help with the healing process.

- Lots of women find perineal bathing with warm water really comforting.
- Lavender oil has been clinically proven to help with perineal healing and to reduce redness. In one study, women got the best results (reduced redness) from regular bathing with lavender oil for the first 10 days after

birth. If you want to try lavender oil for perineal healing, add a drop in 500ml of warm water and pour over your perineum after weeing.

- Ibuprofen and paracetamol taken regularly are a great combination to help you feel comfortable. Try not to take either of these on an empty stomach.
- Pop a clean wet flannel (on a clean plate) in the fridge; you can use it as a nice cold compress for soothing any soreness and swelling.
- A few women have told me about a creative home invention: fill a condom up with water, tie the top and put it in the freezer to make a cooling pad for their perineum. Never put ice directly on the skin as this can give you a 'cold burn' so you can make a hole in the sticky part of a pad and slide it in there.
- Sit on nice comfy cushions or on your side to take the pressure off your perineum.
- Wear the most comfortable clothes ever! Loose, cotton and as open as possible to allow air flow.
- Pour a jug of warm water as you wee or get a wet flannel and wring it out over you as you wee – it can help take any sting out.

YOUR POSTNATAL PELVIC FLOOR

I've always loved France – the food, wine and weather – but the French have got one more thing to boast about. Their fantastic postnatal care. Perineal education is standard care and women are individually assessed on their vaginal strength by a physio, then given tailored exercises for their specific needs, because everyone is different in terms of what they need to do postpartum. We don't offer this in the UK (yet) so it is even more important for you to know how to look after your pelvic floor (see page 126).

It is common to experience incontinence, especially if you are retraining your bladder in the first few days after birth. However, after about a week it is not normal for incontinence to continue. Incontinence is sometimes normalised by adverts and can make bladder leak products seem to be the solution. Rather than use products that only solve the problem not the cause, it is important to look to prevent this all together: incontinence should not be normalised or seen as part of life after birth – incontinence pads are a temporary solution. With the right help and exercises, around 70 per cent of the time those affected can regain strength and correct incontinence.

If your pelvic floor is not re-strengthened after pregnancy, then the pelvic organs can go from feeling heavy to bulging out from their natural position into the vagina (prolapse.) Sometimes a prolapse can be large enough to protrude outside the vagina. Prolapse is reported in almost 50 per cent of women over the age of 50. Take a look at the exercises on page 126, and below.

Yoga pelvic floor exercise

My mum (see page 30) has some yoga exercises that you can easily do at home to help strengthen your pelvic floor; this is useful whether or not you practise yoga.

As the main support of the uterus, the pelvic floor muscles need regular toning and strengthening. This technique will contribute to maintaining a healthy vaginal tone throughout your long-term pelvic health. Give it a go!

This exercise is known as Mula Bandha (mula means 'root' or foundation and bandha means 'lock'). Mula relates to the many blood vessels and nerves passing through and around the pelvic outlet (where your baby passed through during the birth).

In order to use the energy locked in this region, you need to focus on relaxing and then gently lifting the vagina. At first, you will find that it's hard to single out just your vagina and may find yourself lifting your anus and including your urethra all at the same time. With practice, you will be able to isolate just the vagina.

1. Sit cross-legged on a cushion against a wall to support your back.
2. Close your eyes and relax your whole body. Be aware of your natural breath for a few moments. Now, slowly contract your vagina and hold the contraction. Some say to do the contractions on the in breath, some on the out breath. I would say, try which one is best for you. Become totally aware of the physical sensation. Contract your vagina a little tighter but keep the rest of the body relaxed.
3. Then relax the muscles slowly and evenly. Adjust the tension in the spine to help focus the point of contraction.
4. Repeat 10 times with maximum contraction and total relaxation. The point of contraction is actually just behind the cervix (you can try visualising this).

When you are ready to start exercising it's important to take it easy and accept that you may not be able to do what you could right away. But, with a bit of practice and patience you will be able to get your fitness back. Robyn from @ tennison_fitness has trained hundreds of women and has some top tips below for those of you wanting to get back into the gym as soon as possible:

'Slow and steady most definitely wins the race! Your body has not exercised in 6–8 weeks, let alone the nine months whilst you were pregnant and unable to train "normally". Those fast-paced exercise classes burning lots of calories jumping and running around can be very appealing, but trust me, in the long run you will thank your body for starting at the basics.

'Your pelvic floor health should be your top priority. I always say to my clients to book in with a women's physiotherapist because they can assess internally to see if you have any imbalances, along with your pelvis, hips, glutes and abdominals.

'I would never let any of my postnatal ladies jump, run or carry out advanced ab work (e.g., sit-ups, double leg raises etc) shortly after joining me, especially until they have had a thorough check. There has been so much strain on your hips and abdomen for nine months, along with birth, that these forceful movements can actually be damaging. Even if you feel like your bladder control is fine, you will still have internal weaknesses you may not know about. If you feel like you need some guidance then definitely get in touch with a personal trainer who has experience in training pre-and postnatal women.

'Becoming a new mum is manic, so putting 5–6 gym sessions in your diary every week is not going to be sustainable. Gentle bodyweight home exercises are perfect to start with and more than enough. Short 20–30 minute sessions of glute and core strengthening is a perfect way to start and this way you can slot them into your baby's routine. Grab some small resistance bands and ankle weights and you're good to go!

'Think of your goal. Becoming a new mum is so overwhelming and these days there seems to be a lot of pressure on new mums to 'get back into their favourite pair of jeans'. At the end of the day, your goal should be to make sure your body is healthy and strong for your baby. You may end up skipping an exercise session because you haven't slept a wink the night before, so what? It's life, and there will be plenty more days in the future to train. Your mental, emotional and physical health is more important than having a tiny toned frame. If you're not feeling up to formally exercising, then get out and go for a walk in the fresh air with your baby. Walking is so underrated. I think it's amazing to get out with nature and your newborn baby – it's also a great change of scenery.'

SEX AND YOUR RELATIONSHIP

~~~~

We have already talked about the importance of checking in with your partner, and looking after each other (see page 87). So, now it's time to talk about something I get asked about a lot. Sex. Many women are worried about having sex again. It's okay, you don't need to rush into anything and there is no set amount of time that is 'normal'. Having sex after birth is about you feeling ready. Tell your partner how you feel and what is going on and don't put pressure on yourself or have a time frame in your mind – it is best to remove all expectations. Every woman is different; some women are more focused on feeling physically ready and others need to wait until they are more mentally ready. There may also be differences in women who have had a C-section in comparison to women that have had a vaginal birth.

From a clinical point of view the most important thing is to wait until you have stopped bleeding and make sure any wounds have healed. I usually tell women to have a look and feel themselves before they get intimate with anyone else. That way you will be so much more confident and relaxed in the bedroom. If you have a feel and something is sore you can get this checked out first; you may be given some exercises or advised to massage any scar tissue to help that area become comfortable. You may notice that you feel different but your partner probably won't even notice.

The first few times you have sex after birth, use a water-based lubricant, because there is a sudden drop in oestrogen after the delivery of the placenta; you can get quite dry, so it will make sex feel better for you. Doing your pelvic floor exercises is an essential part of improving your sex life after birth, so get going with them as soon as you feel able to (see page 126).

You also need to make sure that you use contraception. It is a myth that you can't get pregnant if you are breastfeeding. My little brother is proof of that ... if you do want to have another baby, particularly if you have had a C-section, it is a good idea to wait until your baby is a year old so that your body has had time to heal and restore. Of course, women have babies sooner and surprises happen, but in order for your body to fully recover and heal a year is a good amount of time to wait.

MUSCLE SEPARATION

It's common for the two muscles that run down the middle of your stomach to separate in pregnancy. The medical term for this is diastasis recti and the amount of separation varies significantly. It happens because as your baby grows your uterus pushes the muscles apart and they become longer and weaker. The majority of women don't notice any problems as this happens in pregnancy, but some might notice a small bulge down the front of their bump.

NHS guidelines recommend a simple technique that you can do at home to check muscle recovery. Do this regularly to check that the gap is gradually decreasing. The separation between your stomach muscles will usually go back to normal by the time your baby is eight weeks old.

1. Lie on your back with your legs bent and your feet flat on the floor.
2. Raise your shoulders off the floor slightly and look down at your tummy. Using the tips of your fingers, feel between the edges of the muscles, above and below your belly button. See how many fingers you can fit into the gap between your muscles.

If the gap is still obvious at eight weeks, the muscles may still be long and weak and this can put you at risk of back problems. Your GP can refer you to a physiotherapist, who will give you some specific exercises to do, or if you prefer you can self-refer and go private.

PROTECTING YOUR POSTURE

Back pain is so common after you have had a baby, but it doesn't have to be, and it can be prevented by doing a few simple things. To help look after your back you need to start by thinking about your posture. If you are breastfeeding, be conscious of your posture as you will probably be sitting in the same position for quite a while. You may feel like you don't want to disturb your baby, especially when they are still trying to get the hang of it, so if you settle into a good posture before you start a feed, you'll avoid this dilemma all together.

I have seen so many women sat feeding in awkward positions, and when I ask 'how's the feeding going?' they respond with, 'great, she's been latched on for ten minutes' and I think, you've held that position for ten minutes! Your poor neck and back! Of course, she is focused on and excited by the fact the baby is feeding well, but this isn't sustainable for her. Accommodating your own needs and getting comfortable before a feed will help protect your back for the future. Here are a few tips:

- You need support to hold your baby while you feed, especially when they are very young. You can use a pillow or large cushion. There are loads on the market and if you have a pregnancy pillow this may double up as a feeding pillow, or just use one from home. Supporting baby on a pillow means you don't have to bend over, and can bring 'baby to breast' more easily.
  - Observe how you are sitting when you are feeding; this is important for both breast- and bottle-feeding mums. Try to think from day one how you are using your body. How are you holding your baby? Are you mainly using your arms? Shoulders? Where's the weight being distributed mostly? Are you twisting and turning? These considerations alone can really reduce long-term problems and pain.
  - As a general rule, have a couple of places set up where you have thought about your posture so you can feed your baby where you are comfortable and supported upright. These places need to be slightly different so that you are using your body in different ways and don't get any repetitive strain injuries.

After having a baby there is general weakness in the abdominal muscles that support your lower back. One of the best things you can do is start moving gently. Your body is in a recovery process so you need to take it easy and be gentle but you need to move the spine, neck and the shoulders. We are able to move because our joints produce fluid which is similar to a lubricant and this keeps things moving. The more we move during the day the more joint lube

HOW ARE YOU HOLDING YOUR BABY?

Take a moment to think about how you carry, burp and cuddle your baby. Do you hold your baby with the same arm or on the same side all the time? For example, so many women only use one shoulder to burp their baby. Try to alternate so that one arm and shoulder aren't always under strain. This is especially important as your baby grows and gets heavier. Try to get into a habit early on of using both sides of your body evenly; think balance. When it comes to picking your baby up, try to avoid bending over because the weight sits in your lower back. Instead, bend your knees to help you lift the weight of your baby.

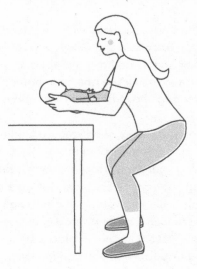

Your baby is only going to grow, get bigger and heavier so it's best to get into good habits when they're small and light. Always think about your body and how you can protect it.

is created at night. It also helps to reduce inflammation. Like most things in the body, it adopts a kind of cycle dependent on the environment. The more movement, the more your body adjusts, the easier it becomes.

YOUR AMAZING 'MUMSTINCT'

One of the biggest tips I can give you in the time after birth is to trust your inner voice, your 'mumstinct'. The best way to be in tune with your instincts is if you're resting and recovering, rather than always 'doing'. I'm sure you've had those random thoughts when you're in the shower, changing the bed sheets or making a cuppa. Thoughts that lead to a realisation or an important decision. Many scientists, leaders and CEOs say some of their very best ideas or discoveries come when doing mundane tasks. That's because they're not 'doing', as such, they're in tune with themselves. Suddenly the answer comes from uninterrupted intuition. All new mums have mumstinct, and it works best when you have the opportunity to tune into it like a radio frequency, cutting out most other noise.

My friend told me: 'Marie, that's nonsense. I knew nothing. I had my first baby at 40, I worked hard all my life in senior roles but I didn't know what to do. I had no such thing as mumstinct.' When we dug a little deeper, she said she was replying to a work email within an hour of giving birth and she was worrying about a project that needed following up on. Of course, she felt like she 'knew nothing'; her brain was full of doing, completing tasks and was unable to tap into her intuition.

THE MUMSTINCT

'I honestly thought this was a crock of shit when I heard people saying, "It'll just kick in!"

'But honestly, it's so true. For me, it didn't happen straight away; you are just working out what this baby is all about and to be fair, you're worried about everything. Even now I still put my hand on his chest to make sure he's breathing. I'm the type of person that needs an answer for everything:

'"Why is he fighting sleep?"

'"Should we be swaddling?"

'"Why won't he take a dummy?"

'As soon as I stopped worrying, my mumstinct kicked in. You literally just know when something is and isn't right.'

Nadia, first-time mum

The other thing you need to try and accept as soon as possible is that there are many ways of doing things, and almost everyone will have an opinion on the decisions all mums need to make, whether it's about sleeping, eating, teething, swaddling, weening and using a dummy or not. From day one, remember that you and your situation is unique to you, and you are the boss. The change of attitude and tips you may have got from managing your pregnancy and birth in 'You're a parent not a patient' (see page 32) need to stick with you for as long as possible. Use the BRAIN tool (see page 37) in the postnatal period too – it is timeless.

Try not to overly compare yourself to anyone else. Tune into who you are becoming as a mum, trust yourself and your own instinct. You know what is best for your baby and your family. There will be times when you may need or seek out expert advice or research things to help you make an informed decision, but ultimately all of the decisions motherhood brings are for you to make. Some people love attachment parenting and others like strict routine – both are just styles of parenting. Rather than get hung up on other people's opinions, take ideas, styles and mums' recommendations to create your own way of doing things. Just like when it comes to breast- or bottle-feeding (see page 296) you don't need to pick a team. Treat it a bit like going into a sweet shop and getting a bag of pic 'n' mix. If you and I went in to a shop and got a bag of pic 'n' mix each, we'd come out with different things and we wouldn't think much of it. We like different sweets. So what? Even if we did choose the exact same sweets, in the exact same amount, what would the chances of us blindly choosing the same sweets in the same order be? Minuscule. Try to see your parenting choices like this and trust your mumstinct. Trust that you chose what you liked and what was right for you. As long as you are being safe and responsible, who cares what way round you do things?

People may judge you at times, but that is not your problem, mamma – it's theirs. Offence is something that is taken not given – as hard as it can be try to tell yourself that if anyone makes an unfair or opinionated comment. You are doing your best, making informed decisions for you and your family.

> 'I think it's really important to find a tribe (be it one person or a group) that just get you, don't judge you, are honest and supportive! Even someone who will listen to you moaning on numerous WhatsApp chats about how your baby hasn't done a poo or how you had to bring your baby into your bed last night. Unfortunately, in motherhood, everyone has an opinion ... EVERYONE ... some people make asshole comments but that's because they're assholes. You just keep doing you.'
>
> Nadz, first-time mum

BABY BAMBOO

So many new mums say to me: 'I'm not getting anything done!' It sometimes feels like you're treading water, just keeping your head above the surface in those first few months, but your perception is far from reality. Your body is doing so much internally to recover and readjust. Your constant attention and care for your baby is time-consuming but it is making such a difference. A monk I met in Tibet told me this story about baby bamboo:

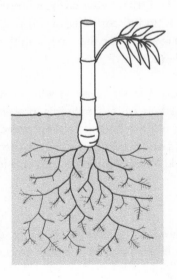

'Bamboo took four years and only grew 3cm. From the fifth year onwards, it grew wildly at a rate of 30cm per day. In just six weeks, it grew to 15 metres. In fact, in the first four years, bamboo has roots extending hundreds of square metres in the soil.'

Like bamboo, your baby takes time to grow and develop properly; it needs to have strong roots. You might not be able to see the extent of the roots but they are larger and deeper than you can imagine.

POSTNATAL NUTRITION

Laura, pre- and postnatal nutritionist (see page 50) is back to explain a bit about postnatal nutrition:

Good nutrition is essential post-birth to help with healing, immunity, balancing mood and sleep. Postnatal is *not* the time to cut out any of the major food groups or severely restrict calories. It is a time of nourishing and respecting our bodies and what they have achieved, rather than punishing them for any new softer spots! The best way to feel healthy postnatally is to eat a well-balanced diet, low in sugar and processed foods, and to eat plenty of vegetables and fruits. I do get mums asking about weight loss so let's talk about it here. Eating a balanced, nutritious diet is best for your body; this naturally leads to a healthy weight. Be aware that 'losing fat' can release toxins into the body which then have to be excreted. This is why, when the time is right, any weight loss must be done slowly and with adequate hydration.

Enjoying warm, well-cooked foods (even in warm weather!) postnatally can help with the easy digestion of the nutrients present, especially iron and zinc, which both help to aid the body's healing process. I often recommend porridge, vegetable soups and broths and slow-cooked recipes such as roasted vegetables or pulled pork. Warm foods are also comforting and so help with our mood too.

Hydrate
Plenty of water is required for successful healing, energy and breastmilk production. Around 2.5 litres a day is a good amount to aim for (roughly

8–10 large glasses). Herbal teas are also good, especially those that contain nettle, fennel and milk thistle, as they can help to boost milk supply if you're breastfeeding.

Good mood food

Our mood can take a serious dip after birth; hormones, lack of sleep and stress can all contribute to feeling blue. There are things that can be done to help boost mood:

- Eat protein with each meal, whether nuts, pulses, dairy or fish and meat. This can help to keep your blood sugar levels stable.
- Include healthy fats such as avocado, nuts, coconut oil, butter and fatty fish such as salmon as they support brain health.
- Include eggs as they are a good source of B vitamins which can help regulate mood.
- Eat regularly throughout the day so you don't get over-hungry. Blood sugar levels need to be kept constant as they are linked heavily to mood.
- Eat a little fermented food each day such as kombucha, kefir and sauerkraut to support gut health.

Many women feel stressed and/or anxious after birth. Stress can deplete nutrients faster than alcohol and smoking combined. The body relies heavily on magnesium and B vitamins in times of stress, so it is important that we replenish these with good food sources which include dark leafy greens, nuts, fish and meats, brown rice, peas and broccoli.

Stress is also one of the main reasons for a drop in breastmilk supply. Aside from trying to reduce the source of stress, you could also include more galactagogues (anecdotal milk-boosting food and drinks) in your day; these include oats, fennel, nutritional yeast (avoid yeast if you have thrush) and flaxseeds.

Consuming plenty of plant foods, packed with antioxidants and polyphenols, helps maintain cell health, which is essential for successful growth and repair. A brilliant way to incorporate these into your diet is through warming soups, or vegetable and berry smoothies. You may need to eat up to an extra 500 k/calories each day if exclusively breastfeeding.

TOP POSTNATAL POWER FOODS

Here are some top foods to include in your postnatal shopping list:

Wholegrains such as buckwheat, oats and brown rice	Nuts
	Offal/Meat
Vegetables	Berries
Pulses	Dark leafy greens and broccoli
Fish and seafood	Eggs
Avocado	

Do you need a multivitamin?

Taking a good-quality multivitamin is recommended as it's difficult to assimilate all our nutrients from the foods we eat due to modern farming techniques (that may strip out some of the nutrients we used to get). There are also specific breastfeeding supplements; pairing them with a high-quality omega-3 algae oil is ideal.

What to avoid

Avoiding processed food, too much sugar, alcohol, caffeine (and definitely smoking) is a great way to help the body's healing process. There is some research that says that having too much sugar may be linked with the onset of UTIs (urinary tract infections) and thrush, both common post-pregnancy. These are what we call 'anti-nutrients' – substances that use up nutrients in the body just to process and eliminate them, whilst providing no nutrition in return.

A healthy gut

Gut health is important for good immunity, successful healing and balancing mood. Maintaining a healthy gut is a major help in terms of regulating inflammation in the body, which is especially important in the fourth trimester when your body is working hard to heal and recover. Good sources of prebiotic foods include bananas, onions, garlic and artichokes. Aim to also include probiotic foods such as live yoghurt, sauerkraut, kimchi and kombucha.

If you or your baby are given antibiotics for any reason, it is helpful to repopulate the gut with good bacteria. At the time of writing, research suggests that our bodies are pretty good at doing this ourselves, and results from probiotic use varies between individuals. If a probiotic supplement is something you want to try, look for ones with at least 30 billion CFU (colony-forming units), containing the Lactobacillus and Bifidus varieties.

Postnatal depletion

Postnatal depletion comes about due to nutrient insufficiency, and leads to symptoms such as forgetfulness, anxiety, debilitating fatigue, insomnia, sensitivity to light and sound, dry skin, softer nails, thinning hair, receding gums and easier bruising. This is not commonly discussed, and Dr Oscar Serrallach, a specialist in postnatal nutrition, is working hard to change this. It's important to know that there are certain autoimmune conditions that can be brought on through pregnancy, such as postpartum thyroiditis. The main message here is that if you're not feeling right, don't just accept it as part of postnatal life – see your midwife or GP for more guidance.

KEY POINTS

- Be patient with your body, it doesn't spring back, but takes time to recover.
- Your pelvic floor has been through a lot, so you need to regain strength, using exercises, as well as rest.
- Incontinence is common but not normal, and can be improved if not totally corrected.
- Don't ignore postnatal pain – see your GP or talk to your midwife.
- Have sex, when you feel ready and comfortable.
- Think about your posture and try to balance weight distribution. Get into good habits while your baby is small and light.
- Your mumstinct is on point, lean on your tribe and ignore opinions you don't need.
- You deserve to eat well and to be well nourished and this will help you to recover and restore during this busy time.

Looking after your newborn

IN THIS SECTION we will cover how to understand your newborn and care for them. We will also look at how to help your baby understand the world, thrive, and get them on their way to become a little confident and independent person.

Even in these early days, your tiny baby is learning what it is like to be human in the world. They are developing a 'sense of self' and it is a very important, magical time. Their nervous system and brain take note of all their experiences to make sense of this strange new world. Some neuroscientists refer to this time as *'unrememberable and unforgettable'*.

HOW TO COMFORT YOUR BABY

In the first few months of life, your baby is still very much an extension of your body and is reliant on you for everything. Newborns have been in darkness, kept warm, cosy and held closely in your womb and now they need to adapt to brightness, a colder temperature and a scarily spacious environment. This takes time, and even though your baby isn't inside you any more, they are still very much an extension of your body.

The time after birth is often called 'the fourth trimester' to recognise that your baby is still dependent on you. It is good to think of your baby as still being a part of you at this time, because they need your body, warmth and comfort – a lot. Please don't worry about 'making a rod for your own back' or holding them too much. Newborn babies need to adapt to life outside the womb gradually and it is okay to hold them, have skin-to-skin and be with them a lot. Research shows that the more babies are held, feel close to someone and feel safe, the more independent they become later on in life.

During the fourth trimester your baby's environment is important, so let's look at three key things you can use to help your baby feel safe and calm:

- Touch, closeness and warmth
- Familiar sounds
- Your face

TOUCH, CLOSENESS AND WARMTH

Touch is crucial for newborns (see page 221). In your or your partner's arms, your baby feels safe and supported – their little muscles relax and their breathing deepens. Holding your baby close, rocking and stroking your baby gives them the best feeling in the world.

What is going on here biologically is communication between your nervous systems through soothing touch. If you are cuddling and stroking your baby in a relaxed state, your baby is more likely to be calm and relaxed as they are learning this from your body. This communication between your bodies works best in skin-to-skin contact and is one of the reasons the World Health Organization recommends skin-to-skin at birth, but also in the weeks following birth. If you watch most babies or young children they will often put their hands up or down mum's top to touch her skin rather than her clothing. Although this isn't always ideal when you're having a civilised conversation (and your baby decides to show everyone your mum tum), it is an expression of instinctive behaviour for babies. You may also have mixed feelings about your mum tum but remember your baby only ever feels and notices the softness, nourishment and warmth of your body. Your baby will never, ever judge your body or how you look because you and your body are such a precious source of comfort.

Your baby's little body can struggle to regulate and generate enough heat, but warm babies do most things better. They feed better, stabilise their blood sugars, heart rate and breathing and can spend their precious energy resources on growing and developing. The perfect place for your baby to be kept warm is in skin-to-skin with you, your partner, birth partner or relative.

REBIRTHING

'When you are 4–5 weeks into your recovery and any stitches are healing well, run a lovely warm bath and, if safe to do so, place candles around the bathroom. Then get into the bath with your baby. This is such a lovely thing to do, kind of like a 'rebirthing', if you will. The baby will love it as the environment is dark, warm and they are in the warm water ... what's not to love?!'

Samantha Pantlin, The Naked Midwives

There are also long-term benefits of touch. It has been shown that lots of physical contact increases brain development in the first six months of life. When studied long-term, evidence of improved cognitive ability was shown at eight years of age, compared to a baby who has received limited physical interaction.

FAMILIAR SOUNDS

Newborns have been very used to hearing the sound of your heartbeat, your digestive system and your voice. Your baby will recognise and prefer your voice at birth to any other. Talking to your newborn helps to calm and comfort them as well as readying them for future language acquisition. Although muffled, babies can hear all sorts of sounds while in the womb. Having the TV on or playing white noise is often comforting for newborns, as they will recognise it from their time with you in the womb.

I know it doesn't always look like it, but your baby is listening to everything you're saying and is paying attention to your voice. Chat away to your baby when you're changing their nappy and going about your day, tell them what you're doing, because they will go on to make the association between specific words and what is happening as they grow. Language is such a huge part of our self-expression and your baby learns so much from your voice, your expressions and your use of language.

Some studies have shown that children in families from disadvantaged backgrounds hear around 600 words per hour on average, whereas children from wealthier backgrounds can hear up to 2,100 words per hour. The most encouraging thing from these findings is the fact that the financial situation is not always what gives children from wealthier backgrounds an advantage. It's the *amount* of interaction they get, and that is free.

WHOOSHING SOUNDS

During pregnancy the sound of your blood whooshing around your body is really loud to a baby, and it is there all the time. Babies are used to sound, and silence can be unnerving to them. Noise can help calm babies down, especially sounds that mimic the whooshing of the womb and this is probably why parents instinctively say shhh to calm a crying baby.

YOUR FACE

Research has proven time and time again that newborns are naturally drawn to faces. For your baby, the world is initially a little out of focus and more difficult to work out, but they can start to recognise your face from as early as three weeks old, so get up close to your baby's face and become recognisable. It is amazing that they have such a strong preference for something they have never seen before!

I was driving along the motorway once thinking about how mind-blowing tiny humans are and what it's like to be a newborn baby, when something suddenly occurred to me. They have never ever seen one of the most important things in our lives. A face. I started to think about all the babies that I have held up close and inspected and watched them gaze at me and my face – until their mum spoke. Then I was less interesting. Babies will often sit and stare at their mums – almost as though they are thinking 'so you're the face of my whole world'.

After my motorway realisation I researched their ability to recognise their mums further, and found an experiment that made me cry (happy tears though!). Are you ready? In Scotland, two new mums that had similar hair and skin colour were asked to sit next to each other behind a clear plastic screen to mask their smell. Their newborn babies (only four days old) were brought into the room separately and held 30cm away from the women's faces. An independent observer watched as the babies looked from one woman to the other before eventually fixating on one woman. Both babies appeared to know who their mum was and gazed at her with adoration. Heart-melting!

I am asked about bonding by a lot of mums in the first few weeks, especially if they are worried that they are not bonding with their baby. This worry is often linked to eye contact and facial expressions. It's normal not to get much eye contact or real interaction before the first six weeks because babies don't have good control over their eye coordination and see the world in more of a 2D-effect. It's not until around six to eight weeks that babies start to become more expressive, maintain eye contact or smile. As they grow, they quickly learn how to control their face more and what these facial expressions mean, but in those first six weeks they are looking, learning and taking it all in.

Human biology and genetic predisposition lay the foundations for cognitive development (thinking ability.) Babies are such adaptive little creatures and really thrive in positive, stimulating and fun environments; they love and look for patterns from birth. Simple things like smiling and interacting through body language helps them learn and understand things for themselves. It's not until 18 months to two years of age that they develop a sense of self but as newborn studies have consistently shown they will turn their heads to look at face-shaped patterns, and normal faces over faces where the position of the features has been distorted. They also spend longer looking at them. It is as though they are born with an innate face detector and the most interesting face of all to them is yours, mamma.

It might take several weeks for you to get the type of human interaction that you need to feel rewarded and reassured that you are doing all the right things. In between that time just know how special you are, how important your touch, voice and your face are to your newborn. It won't be long before you'll get those smiles, gargles and more back from your interactions. Know that nothing is going to waste and all of your attention is being absorbed into that (deliciously smelling) little head.

A HEALTHY NEWBORN

At your postnatal appointments or home visits, midwives do a basic and easy assessment of your newborn by looking at these key things. All of these give us a good picture of how well a newborn baby is:

- Does the baby look well 'perfused'? This meaning are they a good colour.
- Are they warm? We touch the tummy and back of the neck – not the hands and toes – to check core temperature.
- Are they weeing and pooing regularly? See page 302 for more on baby poo.
- Does the cord stump look okay? Or is it smelly and red?
- Are they alert and awake at times during the day?
- Is baby waking for feeds and feeding well?
- Are they responsive to being disturbed?
- Do they have good muscle tone?

A further word on skin colour. When your baby is inside you, they have a high red blood cell count to keep hold of as much oxygen as possible. They break down these red blood cells after birth but the by-product of the breakdown is bilirubin, which can cause jaundice. Sometimes jaundice comes and goes, and in some lights a baby can look quite yellow, but in others they can look fine. Babies that feed well generally 'flush out' any jaundice themselves through feeding, weeing and pooing. Your midwife will check for jaundice and keep an eye on bilirubin levels with a special monitor (if needed) but if you are ever worried about your baby's colour between visits you can always call your midwife.

SECOND NIGHT SYNDROME

I wouldn't be surprised if you have never heard of 'second night syndrome'. Most new parents have a pretty tough night of their baby being restless in that first week after birth, and it's usually on the second night. It's not a real syndrome, don't worry, more of a figure of speech generated from the constant waking, crying and needs of a newborn.

There's a theory, not scientifically proven, that during the first 24 hours, babies fall into a deep sleep after the effort and stress that birth can bring, and when they wake up they become more aware that life as they knew has gone, and they feel hunger for the first time. This new supercharged environment, with sensory overload, is a lot to take in. There's also another theory that the regular need for comfort and feeding is a newborn baby's way of making sure they're on the breast more, so that your body can start making lots of milk. Very frequent feeding is thought to help your milk 'come in', which is usually day three to five. You have milk there but it is a different kind of milk (colostrum, see page 288) and the frequent feeding helps your long-term milk supply. An unsettled newborn is not a reflection of you not having enough milk or your parenting. It is normal newborn behaviour.

Here are some of the things to help keep everything calm and to carry on:

- Have skin-to-skin contact with your baby – research shows this reduces crying. They may cry louder and more angrily as you undress them because they are trying to communicate: 'No I want warmth and comfort! Why aren't you listening?' When you get to skin-to-skin they should calm down.
- White noise, background noise or playing them music you listened to during pregnancy can help babies to settle.
- Don't have too many visitors on day one. All those different voices and smells can be an overwhelming experience for a newborn. Whilst they are adjusting to life outside the womb, being passed around can be stressful. Let your baby get used to their new surroundings gradually and get comfort from the people and smells they already know.

YOUR BABY'S FEELINGS

~~~~~

No matter how responsive you are to picking your baby up, sometimes babies will continue to cry. This tends to reach a peak at about six weeks and the sound of your baby crying can be stressful. Frequent crying is not a reflection on your parenting so please don't doubt your parenting ability. You're doing an amazing job of caring for a tiny human who is totally reliant on you.

Newborns are learning what it's like to feel hungry, alone and tired, which is a lot going on. As unnerving as these sensations can be, all you can do is help your baby to learn that they will be relieved and they can trust you. In the postnatal haze, leaving a baby alone to 'cry it out' can be tempting for some parents, but leaving a newborn baby to cry alone *regularly* can also be harmful and stressful. You might have read headlines recently in the media saying that leaving your baby to cry is the 'best' way to get an infant into a sleep routine; this came from a study that did not include babies under seven months old, so it is not relevant to a newborn or any babies under seven months old. Newborns need responsive parenting and it is not advisable to leave a newborn to 'cry it out'.

A newborn baby should be protected from stress as much as possible so that they can spend their energy on development and growth. That said, if you need a short break, which is perfectly reasonable and okay to admit to, by the way, get someone else to take over or leave your baby in a safe place and have a break. It's not realistic for all parents to never put their crying baby down, particularly unsettled or restless babies – you may need a break in order to be the best version of yourself. Having a break is different to using the 'cry it out' method.

If someone else is able to take over – it doesn't really matter who it is as long as they are caring and nurturing – your baby will generally feel less stressed. I have comforted hundreds of babies over the years and most of them soon settle. I don't doubt every single one knew I wasn't their mum, but I was a warm, caring comforter letting the baby know, 'you're safe and I'm listening. It's scary being out here, I know. You're going to be okay.' Ask for help from those you have planned to have around you in those early days (see page 323).

Coping with crying

All babies cry because it is their only form of communication – although I am sure you already gathered that. Some researchers believe that babies are born about three months before they're physically ready to enter the world in order for them to be able to fit through the pelvis, which is why they need so much looking after from you. Some specialists believe that if a human baby were born with the maturity of a chimpanzee, pregnancy would last 17 months ... can you imagine?! This theory is another reason that people refer to the first three months of a baby's life as the fourth trimester (see page 272). Most parents, especially with their first baby, worry when their baby is crying and think they are doing something wrong. The truth is we do not always know or find out why some babies cry more and for longer periods than others. But there are a few common reasons that your baby maybe crying so here is a checklist to go through:

- **Is your baby hungry?** Young babies are hungry very frequently, sometimes every two hours.
- **Do they have a wet or dirty nappy?** This can be an uncomfortable sensation, so check and change regularly.
- **Wind?** It's a myth that breastfed babies don't need winding; they can do, even from a young age, so try gently winding by holding them up near one shoulder, and use circular motions with a flat hand and then pat.
- **Too hot/too cold?** The ideal room temperature is 16–20°C.
- **Are they startled?** Was there a sudden noise? Or maybe they suddenly realised they are separate from you and need a cuddle.
- **Colic?** This usually affects babies from three weeks to four months and it is quite common. Babies with colic will usually cry excessively for no apparent reason, go red in the face, and bring their knees up to their chest. It is a bit of an umbrella term for a range of possible causes although the word colic comes from the Greek 'kolikos', meaning of the colon. It is thought to be caused by cramps from wind, intolerances, feeling stressed, growth of the immature digestive system and/or muscle spasms. Gentle baby massage (if you have learned this) when your baby is happy and alert can help. There are also some medications available to buy but ask your midwife or health visitor about these first.

- **Tired?** Sometimes it's not as easy as you may think it is for them to sleep. Some babies get over-tired or over-stimulated, especially if they have just had different people handling them.
- **Something else** could be causing discomfort, like a thread wrapped on the toe or uncomfortable clothing – do a quick check.

Seek help from your midwife or health visitor if you are worried about your baby's crying or signs of distress.

SLEEP AND ROUTINE

To be honest, there is no getting away from sleepless nights at first, but I promise it gets better. Within the fourth trimester you can't have or make any 'bad' sleep habits, and you can't spoil a newborn. Also, your baby has no real concept of day and night yet. Their circadian rhythm is immature, meaning their melatonin (the sleepy hormone) production is a bit all over the place. Newborns want to feed more at night and that is instinctive to them (more on this on page 289). As mentioned, they are still very much an extension of your body and will want to be on you, feeding, or with you a lot of their waking hours. This is normal newborn behaviour, however, there is no harm in implementing an easy routine early on if you want to. In fact, some research suggests that a flexible routine for babies under eight weeks reduces crying.

By routine I don't mean any form of sleep training or rigidity. Trials have shown that sleep training doesn't work in babies under three months old anyway. What we do know is that babies like patterns, habits and cues. You can keep a routine very low effort by sticking to just doing a few simple things every night, perhaps skin-to-skin in dim lighting, playing the same calming song, followed by a feed then bed. When you attend to them during the night, just turn on a dim night light rather than the main bedroom light, too. This starts to introduce the idea of a 'night-time' routine.

You can also introduce a lot of daylight in the morning, and say 'good morning' every morning. Studies found that babies exposed to more natural light in the day slept better at night.

An early routine works for some mums and others hate the idea of it or feel like it is added unnecessary pressure. Whatever you decide, don't expect too much too soon. Do what is most suitable for you and your family. Trust your mumstinct here and have confidence that you are doing what is right for you.

THE NEWBORN BRAIN

A young baby's brain is like a sponge soaking up experiences and recording patterns. The structure of the infant brain is highly complex and designed to be ready to learn. We are born with all the neurons we will ever need, that's around 86–100 billion, but what babies need to do is make synaptic connections and strengthen pathways between the neurons. As newborns make those connections, their ability to use particular areas of the brain start to develop; it's a bit like dot-to-dot. From birth to age three years is the fastest rate of brain development in the entire human life span. Up to 65 per cent of their energy intake is spent on the brain, compared to around 20 per cent in adults, and within the first year of life a baby's brain doubles in weight. There's an awful lot going on in there!

The pathways that are used the most are strengthened and the ones that aren't used die off. This process is called 'pruning'. If you regularly show your baby love, respond to their needs, and build trust, their brain will remember those experiences forever. One of the keys to helping your baby make connections is simply love and responsive parenting. Sue Gerhardt has a whole book dedicated to this called *Why Love Matters*.

We are emotional creatures, dependent on feelings. Newborns don't have mature thought processes yet; they go more by feeling. The phenomenon known as 'failure to thrive' that you may have heard of was discovered by very cruel experiments on monkeys. I really don't condone what researchers did, but the only understanding we can take from this research was that primates need to feel comfort and attachment in order to *thrive*, not just survive. We also know that babies are seriously damaged for the rest of their lives if they are not attached to, or feel love from, a human. Those are extremes but they show how our very existence as humans is based on feelings, not just thoughts. Just

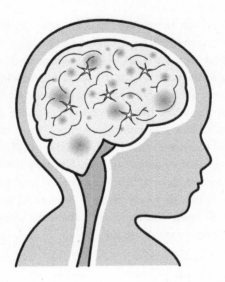

like monkeys, human babies thrive with emotional attachment and bonding — babies need to be dependent before they can be independent.

'Affection is like the electrical tape that bonds neurons together. Once the connection among neurones is established, affection comes in and makes the bonds so strong it can never be undone.'

— **DR FLAVIO CUNHA**

Scientists are now discovering the huge impact environment has on infant development. Many experts agree that you cannot judge anything separate from its environment, and epigenetics (additional information layered on top of the sequence of letters that makes up DNA) mean certain genes can be switched on and off. In other words, the environment your baby grows up in significantly influences their understanding of the world and their personality.

Your baby has so much to learn. We take for granted that when someone jumps up in the air gravity will bring them back down. Your baby doesn't understand the simplest, general rules of the universe and won't do for a while. Nothing is predictable yet and this can be a bit overwhelming at times. Plus, things change extremely quickly. For example, your baby's head circumference suddenly increases in size when they are going through a growth spurt, which explains why their behaviour can change so much from one day to the next. Just when you thought you have nailed this parenting stuff, their needs change. Don't worry about momentary setbacks; they happen often, especially where sleep and feeding are concerned. Ask any parent and they will tell you it's just a phase and there are so many phases! Some will feel good, some not so good, and they will keep changing with minimal to no warning. Always remember you are doing an amazing job.

KEY POINTS

- Your baby's brain is ready to learn and loving comfort helps to shape it.
- Skin-to-skin = communication between nervous systems.
- Leaving a baby alone to cry is stressful for your baby.
- If you need help, ask for help and get someone to take over. Your baby will be just fine with someone else holding them.
- Babies need their dependence to be met before they can learn to be independent.

What you *really* need to know about breastfeeding

BREASTMILK HAS BEEN evolving for millions years and provides optimum nutrition for your baby. But facts about breastfeeding and the phrase 'breast is best' isn't going to help you at 3am when you're tired, sore and shuffling over to your hungry baby. Perhaps it's time we abandon simple slogans and focus on *how* to, rather than *why* to. It is impossible for me to tell you everything you may need to know about breastfeeding in this section as there are so many variables involved, so what I have done is focus on the key things that are evidence-based and recommended by most professionals. It is also important to start by saying that there is a huge difference between reading about breastfeeding and actually experiencing it. It is different for every single woman: some take to it immediately, while others struggle immensely. It's a very natural thing but it doesn't always come naturally.

The most important message to take from this section is to remember that millions of women breastfeed healthy babies and millions of women also formula-feed healthy babies. I'm not going to sugar-coat how hard breastfeeding can be at times. Britain's low breastfeeding rate is not linked to women not wanting to breastfeed. It's often down to lack of support, unrealistic expectations of postnatal women, and a lack of education surrounding normal behaviour for breastfed babies.

We naturally want to do the very best for our children, so we give it our best, but it is important to remember that *your* mental health is paramount. Your baby needs you to make the choices that are right for you – not right for anyone else – including social-media influencers, the press and any other mums. Like birth, you can have a plan for breastfeeding, but you may have to deviate from it and if you need to, it's okay. Please, please, please do not feel guilty if you give your baby formula for whatever reason. You are doing the best for you and your baby and if that means formula-feeding, so be it, you are not failing anyone. No guilt attached!

That said, I urge everyone to give breastfeeding a go. There are so many well-known health benefits for your baby, such as boosting their immunity, and reducing the risk of asthma and diabetes and many more. Just breastfeeding your baby even once can be helpful, especially if it is the first feed because this helps to colonise the gut (see page 287).

So many mums tell me that being able to bond with their baby is the best feeling in the world, especially when they are around six months and life is so busy. Breastfeeding gives you the time to be alone with your baby, somewhere peaceful – just bonding.

If you choose not to breastfeed at all then bottle-feeding is just as good of an opportunity to bond with your baby. Keep them lovely and close throughout feeds so they can really see your facial features. In those early weeks try to keep feeds quite intimate and private by only allowing a small number (you and your partner ideally) to feed your baby. This protected time and feeds don't need to go on forever; the early weeks are the most important.

BREASTFEEDING AND IMMUNITY

Thanks to a few badass evolutionary biologists like Katie Hinde, I am able to share some cutting-edge facts about how breastmilk actually works and what it does for your baby's immune system so that you can make your own informed choice.

A well-functioning immune system is vital for overall health throughout life and only fairly recently are scientists and doctors really starting to understand the role of the immune system, inflammation and gut health. A newborn baby needs help to build their immune system right from the start. While newborns arrive equipped with some natural immunity, they still need a significant amount of help to build on this foundation.

Breastfeeding helps build your baby's immune system and gut colonisation. The nutritional and immunological components of breastmilk change daily, according to the specific, individual needs of your baby. Some fairly new research has come out that tells us that when your baby is on the breast, some of your baby's saliva is suctioned into your nipple so you can adapt your milk especially for your baby to help them fight specific infections.

> 'In 2015, researchers found that the mixture of breastmilk and baby saliva – specifically, baby saliva – causes a chemical reaction that produces hydrogen peroxide that can kill staph and salmonella.'

> Katie Hinde, TED Talk 'What we don't know about mother's milk'

As well as fighting potential infection, as Katie Hinde mentions in her TED Talk, quoted above, breastmilk contains the perfect combination of proteins, fat, carbohydrates and nutrients that your baby needs. It also contains sugars called oligosaccharides that are unique to human milk. Your baby can't digest these oligosaccharides and they only exist to feed the microbes in your baby's digestive system.

The latest research into babies born via C-section and their gut health showed some interesting findings. Previous studies have been fairly consistent in their findings showing that babies born via C-section develop a different gut microbiome compared to babies that are born vaginally. These differences have been linked to increased chances of C-section babies developing autoimmune diseases like asthma and eczema. However, the most recent research (at the time of writing) shows a different picture. The research took poo samples from 596 babies born in UK hospitals. Samples were collected in the weeks following birth and then again between 6–9 months old. They found that 80 per cent of the C-section babies had hospital-acquired bacteria in their gut at birth, compared to 50 per cent of babies born vaginally. But, those differences largely disappeared in the samples from babies aged 6–9 months. All of the babies studied were healthy.

This is in line with previous research, and also tells us that, yes, there is a difference in the microbiome when you can compare C-section babies to vaginally born babies. But there is no evidence from this study that this has implications for long-term health. It is more likely that many other factors, like breastfeeding and early life exposures, play a large part in the microbes that colonise a baby's gut.

COLOSTRUM IS KEY

The first milk you'll produce is called colostrum and it is low in fat but high in carbohydrates and protein, making it quickly and easily digestible. It also contains Lactoferrin – this stuff is hardcore when it comes to fighting infection and protecting the gut. So, even if you breastfeed for a few days, and get the colostrum in, that really helps your baby. There are far more white cells in colostrum than in the milk that comes later on and it has the most amount of vitamins in it, particularly vitamin A (immune-boosting) and vitamin K (haemorrhage-preventing). The highly complex components of colostrum also help develop immature organs. If you are struggling with feeding and did manage to harvest some colostrum, just that tiny 1ml can make a difference too (see page 26 for more on how to harvest colostrum).

Now you're up to date with the latest science about what breastmilk does, let's get on to the tips that should help you establish breastfeeding.

GETTING OFF TO A POSITIVE START

Skin-to-skin contact at birth is one of the main factors that will contribute to you meeting your breastfeeding goals. Although there is plenty of research to suggest this, the benefits go beyond any scientific explanation, and when you're in skin-to-skin contact with your baby you'll know just what I mean by this. If you plan to breastfeed, ideally, you should try to feed within the first six hours of birth. Your body needs to get the message that you are breastfeeding and a cocktail of hormones will take over to enhance your milk production –

your body is on the look-out for these signals more attentively in the first six hours. If your baby needs to go to special care and you can't put them on the breast within the six-hour window, then you can hand-express because it's the early and frequent extraction of milk that helps to establish supply. Your midwife can help you to do this.

UNDERSTANDING NEWBORN FEEDING BEHAVIOUR

Understanding normal newborn behaviour plays a huge part in a woman's confidence around breastfeeding. I think it will help to know that your newborn baby's tummy is about the size of a marble, which is why they need **very regular feeding**. This is normal so ignore anyone that tells you their baby 'sleeps through the night' – newborns aren't designed to do that and most breastfeeding mums are up every couple of hours to feed. Frequent feeding and cluster feeding (where your baby wants to feed at close intervals) are both normal behaviours for most breastfed newborns. If you supplement with a bottle at this time and don't stimulate your breasts regularly, it can disrupt breastfeeding. Your supply can be reduced and (if given a lot of formula at one time) your baby's stomach can be stretched from a formula feed, making it more difficult for you to then satisfy your baby's feeding needs. Those first few weeks of breastfeeding are *intense* but it really does get easier after that.

For breastfeeding your baby needs:

- To be close to your body and to have their head, shoulders and body in a straight line.
- To have their chin and lower lip touching the breast first. Your nipple needs to be near their nose, rather than the mouth at first.
- To have their head free to tilt back. Try not to hold your baby's head; support the shoulders and neck but avoid pushing their head.
- To have their mouth wide open – looking like they are about to yawn.
- To take a large mouthful of the breast tissue – not just the nipple.
- Have more areola (the small bumps around your nipple) above their top lip than below.

BABY-WEARING AND BREASTFEEDING

Baby-wearing (see page 131) is great for encouraging breastfeeding and bonding because it provides easy access to the breast for your baby and easy access to the top of your baby's scrumptiously smelling head. You can also take your baby out and about hands-free or pop them in your sling if you need to get on with something else at home. If you are using a sling, make sure you do so safely. Put the baby in an upright position with a straight, flat back and check that their head is supported. Keep close enough to kiss and in view at all times.

THE ROOTING INSTINCT

Your newborn has a 'rooting reflex' and may start looking for food (this usually happens within the first hour of birth). They often start by rubbing their head around on your chest which marks their smell and works like a sat-nav for their next meal. Later on they follow the sat-nav and remember they have been there before and fed. So, as strange as this sounds, try not to wash this off until the next feed after birth (usually that's only a few hours but if you want to wash it off – go for it).

YOUR FAMILIAR FACE

Initially, your baby doesn't yet have the ability to see or focus all that well; by keeping your baby close, they can start to recognise your face. Research has now shown that this can happen as early as three weeks old. If you are bottle-, syringe- or cup-feeding, try and have your baby nice close to you for that early bonding and facial recognition. This reduces cortisol levels (stress levels) in your baby and makes them feel protected and calm by being able to recognise a familiar face.

IS YOUR BABY GETTING ENOUGH MILK?

～～～

A baby that is alert, feeding well, and has wet and dirty nappies is usually a well-fed baby who is getting enough food. Sometimes there can be a focus on baby's weight and it is normal for exclusively breastfed babies to lose weight in the first few days and therefore be below birth weight at their day five weigh-in. If your midwife is concerned about your baby's weight loss (s)he will calculate it (generally, it should be less than 10 per cent weight loss; it is commonly 7–8 per cent of birth weight according to recent research) and ensure that your baby does not need any further input from paediatricians or a feeding plan. When assessing if your baby is getting enough it is best to focus on your baby's behaviour and what's coming out the other end. Are they alert and waking, feeding well, weeing and pooing? That's great! On that note, don't be alarmed if you have a little girl and find some mucus vaginal discharge that's blood streaked. This is called pseudo-menstruation and is caused by her having been exposed to your hormones. However, if you chose not to have vitamin K you need to let your midwife know as soon as possible.

MAKING BREASTFEEDING WORK FOR YOU

～～～

As mentioned, although natural, breastfeeding does not come naturally to many new mums. Making breastfeeding as comfortable as possible gives you a better chance of reaching your breastfeeding goals and continuing. Here are some tips that have worked for the women in my care; you can get some of this before baby arrives, or get your partner to pop out and buy them now, if you need! Support from other women can also be incredibly helpful, particularly in the early days.

- Invest in a few breastfeeding bras if you're planning on exclusively breastfeeding for six months (the recommended advice). Your breasts get swollen and tender so get one that opens completely when you take the clip down. You don't want any restrictive straps. Try them on before your baby is here, so you know it's easy to use and comfy.
- Breastfeeding pillows are great for supporting the weight of your baby and can help raise your baby to the height you need to bring baby to breast, without you bending forward.

- A natural nipple balm, you can start using this before baby arrives to prepare your nipples, and use after each feed (see below and page 114).
- Invest in a decent breast pump. There are some serious advances in technology and you can get hand pumps and electric pumps; there are now even portable pumps on the market that you can wear in your bra! These are great for when you're out and about or planning on going back to work. Pumping can help with supply and can also help give you a break while your partner does a feed. Giving breastmilk in a bottle is only recommended when breastfeeding is well established and some women prefer to not to give their baby breastmilk in a bottle. Do whatever works for you. Get as much free help from the NHS as possible and ask to see a breastfeeding consultant early on, especially if you have flat or inverted nipples. You can absolutely breastfeed but you may need a little more support with attachment so you don't get sore nipples.
- If you give birth in hospital, don't leave until you're happy with your baby's feeding. If you rush home, you'll probably regret it and may need to come back in.
- Join a breastfeeding group either in your community or on social media. Some mums have said that they have found some groups a bit full-on and pressurising, so perhaps see what the vibe is like before baby arrives. If you're reading mostly random rants, leave and look elsewhere. Sling Meets (peer-to-peer support meetings, facilitated by volunteers who are experienced baby-wearers) are great and are around most of the country so have a look into one in your area.
- Watch videos of how to breastfeed online. Most of us have not seen a woman breastfeed; just watching breastfeeding videos will give you a wealth of knowledge.
- Ask someone you feel comfortable with who is currently or has breastfed to help you with tips too. It is great to have real-life support. Other mums who have breastfed will be able to share their tips and help you out.

NIPPLE PAIN

One of the top reasons women stop breastfeeding earlier than they planned is due to nipple pain. Start nipple care early on by using nipple cream after

FEEDING AFTER A C-SECTION

Try different positions to take the pressure off your tummy, like lying on your side or with your baby's head in your hand, spine on your forearm and their feet under your arm. Babies born by C-section may cough up mucus in the first few days (they are clearing their lungs after birth), so your baby may not be interested in feeding for very long. It is important to keep putting your baby to the breast, or express breastmilk, every few hours, so that your body continues to produce milk. Once the mucus has been cleared, your baby should feed more often and for longer.

every feed to help you nipples stay comfortable. If you are in pain it's likely that the latch is not quite right. Try a change of position and make sure you're comfy, re-latch your baby and aim for a deep latch; you want your baby to have a proper mouthful of breast tissue and is not just sucking the end of your nipple. If the pain is so bad that you're dreading the next feed, make sure you get help *right away*; you can always call your community midwife. Some women swear by healing cups (they help to prevent, protect and heal cracked nipples) you can get online and some prefer balms. You may also want to ask about checking for a tongue tie if you have nipple pain and difficulty latching.

HOW LONG DO YOU WANT TO BREASTFEED FOR?

I think it is worth taking a moment to think about how long you would like to breastfeed for, if at all. What are your personal breastfeeding goals? What do you want to achieve on your breastfeeding journey? This choice is your own and *no one* has the right to question or judge you for that. If you plan to breastfeed for months ahead, that goal will take some persistence. One top priority is to encourage and protect a good milk supply. Without a good supply you may not be able to exclusively breastfeed, and there is a critical time you need to pay particular attention to, days three to five. So let's look at this in more detail.

There is a key window of opportunity that affects long-term milk supply. The scientific term for describing this window is lactogenesis I to lactogenesis II; it is when you go from producing colostrum (the first milk you may have leaked or expressed in pregnancy) to the milk you'll produce for the rest of the time you feed your baby. This is your milk 'coming in'.

It's normal to not have a lot 'milk' before day three. Many women say to me, 'I have no milk' around this time, and although it feels like it, it's not the case. You do have milk, it's just a different kind of milk. Ignore the amount in pre-made formula bottles; this isn't a realistic reflection of what your baby needs.

Feeding your baby every few hours is hard work but it is worth persisting for those first five days. If you don't extract milk regularly during this window, your milk supply can be affected. It may sound simple now but it can be hard work and exhausting, particularly when you are already tired and recovering from birth.

To 'extract' milk you can regularly feed, hand-express (see page 26 for how to) and some women choose to pump. If your baby is well and waking regularly for feeds, it is fine to feed on demand, but if you have a sleepy, small or jaundiced baby this is different and you need to either wake them for feeds or protect your own supply by expressing (usually this is if your baby needs to go to SCBU and you are able to put them to the breast) and you will get extra support to do this.

Your body is perfectly designed for breastfeeding, although there are some very rare genetic or health reasons why some women can't breastfeed. Our bodies are very smart; they need to know what is going on so they can make some decisions about investment.

Some women worry about their milk supply and they leave their boobs to fill up thinking that they will make more milk if they do so. This can have the opposite effect as milk production works on a demand/supply basis – the more you give out, the more you need to produce.

Milk contains protein which inhibits milk production so your body knows when to slow down and you will produce less milk if your breasts are too full. So, allowing your breasts to 'fill up' tells your body 'stop making milk, it's not being used'.

PROTECT THIS TIME

You need to focus on feeding until it is established and you feel confident and happy. You may think you want visitors, but this is when your body is really getting into the flow of breastfeeding, so maybe hold off on the visitors if you can until after this window. Your boobs can look up to double the size, become quite sore and you'll probably feel the effects of the new hormonal cocktail emotionally. Most women get teary and can cry for no apparent reason. Don't worry, it should pass (if it doesn't see page 310 for more on postnatal depression). The various hormones released are really special in terms of human biology as you go into lactogenesis II. If you think visitors will help, do what is best for you, but maybe plan to put people on hold while you're at this stage and only have very close family, midwives and doula (if you have one) over.

FOCUS ON YOU

Not so long ago (in terms of human evolution) and today in many parts of the world (see page 254), a breastfeeding mum mainly feeds, feeds, feeds, sleeps, sleeps, sleeps and the partner protects, hunts or shops and feeds the mum. In the Western world, postnatal life can be very different and there's a bit of a disconnection between what mums think they should be doing and what they really should be doing, especially if they have breastfeeding goals. Stay in your little breastfeeding bubble as long as you can, and don't let any external pressures pop it. This new baby zone will only happen a select few times in your life, and many second-time mums say to me that they wish they had been more relaxed first time and just stayed at home and ignored everything else.

If you have home helpers (partner, mum, sister, friend etc.) pre-warn them that you want to breastfeed and will need to just focus on the feeding, recovering, eating and sleeping for the first week or so. Tell them you won't be doing much else other than that, so you'll need them to cook or sort things out at home because feeding your baby and recovering have to come first. We are mammals and if you observe mammals of all types, the early focus on feeding is normal for a new mother and has been for thousands of years. If you try and socialise and fit in with lots of visitors, this can tire you out for feeding, or make you feel you need to skip feeds, just as you are getting the hang of it.

IT DOESN'T HAVE TO BE
ALL OR NOTHING

~~~~

Some women breastfeed for years, some top-up or mix feed their baby, and some breastfeed just for the first few colostrum days. Whatever you do, and why, is not anyone else's business. But women have told me they felt like they needed to pick a team – breast or bottle. No new mum should ever feel like that; if you want or need to give your baby formula for whatever reason then it doesn't mean you have to join the 'other team'. Just do what works for you. If you have long-term breastfeeding goals you now know about the window of opportunity and making sure you protect that, but if you can't or it doesn't go to plan it's okay. Do what you can at the time and if you need to change course then go for it. It doesn't have to be all or nothing, you can create your own feeding plan that works for you and your baby. You're the boss. You really have got this.

'Forget past mistakes. Forget failures.
Forget everything except what you're going to
do now.'

— **WILLIAM DURANT**

KEY POINTS

- Get all the professional help and advice you can, from the NHS, videos, friends and online networks.
- Protect your milk supply – feeding early and feeding often can help.
- If possible, put baby on the breast to get things going within six hours of birth.
- Skin-to-skin contact at birth is key whatever type of birth you have. It significantly increases the success of breastfeeding. If you can't do this at birth do it as soon as possible and for as long as possible.
- The fourth trimester is the time to have all the skin-to-skin time that you can fit in.
- Get comfortable before the feed; it's worth spending time to get it right. You may want something under your arm or shoulder. Being uncomfortable is not only unpleasant it's not sustainable for an entire feed and may lead to back pain.
- Note how well you're both doing by the wet and dirty nappies you're getting; what's coming out reflects what's going in.
- It doesn't have to be all or nothing with breast- and bottle-feeding; do what works for you.

Skincare for baby

NEWBORN SKIN IS beautiful and biologically it is amazing, too. In the womb your baby has been in a controlled environment in amniotic fluid and their skin is a product of that environment at birth. We all know baby's skin is delicate and sensitive but the physiology of the skin is rarely explained, yet how you care for your baby's skin now may have long-term implications. Here we will run through how you can help protect your baby's skin for life.

The skin is the human body's largest organ and is a major defence mechanism. It regulates temperature, acts as a barrier to infection, balances water and electrolytes, stores fat and helps humans to stay warm in the cold. Newborn skin is around five times more absorbent than ours, so rubbing anything on your baby's skin is will be absorbed quickly. Babies are not born with mature skin that functions like ours; it takes at least four weeks to build up protective natural enzymes that help to develop a protective barrier.

Advice to parents on this subject is often inconsistent, which can be a problem. You may see the term 'suitable for newborns' being marketed to you on wash products, but remember that the baby products industry is very competitive and lucrative. Experts agree that no product should be marketed as 'safe for newborns', and even products labelled 'sensitive', 'natural' or 'organic' may still contain ingredients that are potentially harmful.

Below are some key points about your baby's skin:

- Babies are born with an alkaline skin surface; it has an average pH of 6.34 where as an adult's is around 5.5. However, within days, the pH falls to about 4.95 (acidic) forming the 'acid mantle'. This is a fine film that rests on the surface of the skin acting as a protective barrier. Its delicate balance must be maintained if the skin is to achieve an optimum level of protection. There is no evidence to prove the acid mantle exists beyond the first few days, so baby products, soaps or moisturisers cannot 'become' or 'replace' the acid mantle because it is the body alone that produces and maintains it.

- Your baby is born covered in a white, sticky layer, the vernix caseosa (VC). This 'cheesy varnish' is a highly sophisticated bio-film containing a ton of antimicrobial peptides, proteins and fatty acids. These combine to form a protective barrier that is not only antibacterial but also anti-fungal. A recent scientific paper about VC states: 'Studies confirm that maintaining an intact epidermal barrier by minimising exposure to soap and by not removing VC are simple measures to improve skin barrier function.' The World Health Organization adds: 'Lipid-rich vernix is a natural moisturiser and skin cleanser and has wound-healing, anti-infective and anti-fungal properties. Therefore, it is essential that vernix is not removed at birth.' We look at when to wash your baby below (see page 300).
- Overdue babies are sometimes born with dry and cracked skin. This is usually because the VC has already been absorbed. It will usually peel off and leave perfect skin underneath without any help.
- UK rates of childhood eczema are among the highest in the world. The steady rise in infant skin conditions appears to be co-incident with the introduction of manufactured baby products over 50 years ago.

Penelope Jagessar Chaffer has a brilliant TED Talk called 'The Toxic Baby,' and she explains how easy it is to get chemicals into the body via the skin. Penelope explains how we now have 30,000–50,000 more chemicals in our bodies than our grandparents had.

Because newborn skin is so absorbent and vulnerable to damage, I often tell mums, 'If you wouldn't feed it to your newborn then don't put it on their skin'. Unlike organic food, the legal standards for organic and natural cosmetic products aren't quite as tight, so the question of eating it works well when wondering about whether or not you should use it on your newborn's skin. Of course if you have been prescribed something this is different, but in general, that is a good question to consider. To find certified organic products, there are five European certification bodies who've developed the Cosmetics Organic

Standard (COSMOS) to try and standardise organic standards around the world. They have high standards, and to get a COSMOS certification for a product it has to meet strict criteria with guaranteed organic ingredients.

Sharon Trotter is an experienced midwife, mother of five and parenting consultant specialising in breastfeeding and neonatal skincare. She has been published in various peer-reviewed midwifery journals and textbooks regarding neonatal skincare and has a brilliant website called Tipslimited.co.uk for both parents and professionals. There is a wealth of information from her work over the past 35 years on there, from breastfeeding and tongue-tie to twins and travel tips. I read some of her research papers and dropped her an email one day; we have now been in contact over the past few years about neonatal skincare as the amount of products I was seeing coming into hospital for newborns was starting to concern me.

During our conversations, Sharon made a really good point: 'Research has taught us that we now know better exactly how the skin works and why protecting it from day one can, and will, have far-reaching benefits to a child as they grow older. It cannot be looked at in isolation though, so a healthy pregnancy, early skin-to-skin contact and breastfeeding, alongside water-only skincare for at least the first month of life, will all help to protect babies and children from the damaging effects of the modern world and all its dangers.'

After talking to Sharon and looking at the evidence available I have come up a simple list that consolidates the advice to best care for your newborn baby's skin:

- Avoid bathing your newborn for at least the first 24 hours. Wait until their temperature has stabilised or better still, wait until the umbilical cord stump has come off (see page 301).
- Vernix should always be left to absorb naturally. Studies confirm that maintaining an intact epidermal barrier by minimising exposure to soap, and by not removing vernix, are simple measures to improve skin barrier function.
- When bathing or washing, use water only for the first month of life. This may contradict what you read elsewhere, but remember that this approach is recommended by leading health organisations.

- Bathing daily can dry out the skin; bathing two or three times a week is enough.
- Avoid using wash cloths in the first month because they can be too harsh on your baby's skin – use your hands, cotton wool (organic is preferable) or a natural/bamboo sponge instead.
- Ears, nose and eyes should be left alone when washing, and cotton buds avoided. If your baby has sticky eyes talk to your midwife, health visitor or GP before using anything.
- Baby wipes should not be used until meconium has passed. After this, it is best to use wipes that are free from alcohol, parabens, phthalates, artificial colours and perfumes.
- Shampoo is not needed until your baby is around a year old – after this, any shampoo used should be sulphate-free (usually listed as SLS and SLES).
- A thin layer of barrier cream can be used on the nappy area when you feel necessary – ideally free from preservatives, colours, perfumes, and clinically proven to be effective treatment for nappy rash.
- If you would like to massage your baby, the World Health Organization recommends using sunflower oil (not olive oil), and some hospitals recommend grapeseed oil.
- If you decide to use baby skincare products after four weeks make sure that you read the labels carefully. Carry out a patch test before using any new products.

At present, there's no evidence that using washing powders with enzymes (bio powders) or fabric conditioners will irritate your baby's skin, but knowing what we do about the sensitivity of neonatal skin it makes sense to reducing chemical exposure if you can. One alternative is to use bicarbonate of soda in your wash; it won't cause harm if the clothes are on a hot wash and kills bacteria.

CORD STUMP CARE

When we clamp and cut the cord we leave a little stump that stays attached to your baby for up to ten days, but it usually falls off sooner. You should avoid handling this little stump, but it is fine to touch it if you need to, and it won't hurt to move because there aren't any nerve cells in the cord. Always make sure you've got clean hands before touching the cord as there's a risk you can introduce infection. It is natural and normal for it to shrivel up, going from white and floppy to brown and crispy; one woman told me it reminded her of a pork scratching and now I can't get that analogy out of my head when I see a dried-up cord.

Below are some key things you need to know about cord care. If it smells or there's redness around the area, ask your midwife to have a look ASAP because it could be a sign of infection.

- Keep the area around the cord clean and dry; check during nappy changes.
- The nappy should be folded back at each change so the stump is outside of the nappy until the cord falls off. This helps it to air dry. Poo explosions mean a risk of contamination of the cord if it's left inside the nappy.
- Only use water and cotton wool to clean the area if dirty.
- Avoid using antiseptics unless it has been advised to you by a paediatrician.
- Avoid bathing your baby fully until the separation of the umbilical cord is complete so you don't disrupt the flora at the base of the cord and potentially hinder the natural process of cord separation.

YOUR BABY'S BUM

Being concerned about what comes out of your baby's bum must be instinctive, because all new mums are fascinated by their baby's little bums and poo. Research backs up my thoughts here. Scientists found that new mums prefer the smell of their own baby's poo to that of any other babies! Some mums have confessed that the smell of other babies' nappies make them gag but their own baby's poo is a guilty pleasure. It's unlikely that anyone else will admit that to you, so I thought I would – it's normal to like the smell of your baby's poo.

In the first few days after birth your baby will pass some strange-looking stuff called meconium. It's not like normal poo because it is just the contents of what your baby could swallow in your tummy, that's delicious things like epithelial cells, lanugo, mucus, amniotic fluid, bile and water – appetising! Meconium is a bit like Marmite – dark, sticky and difficult to get off – so try to change your baby as soon as they have pooed this 'mec' (as midwives call it) because it's easier to get off whilst it's wet and sticky. You'll probably get about two of these mec nappies per day, maybe more.

Around day three or four you may notice a slight change in poo colour as it becomes greener. It's a sign your baby is digesting milk well. Yay!

By day five you should have noticed another change – your baby starts to pass yellow/light green 'English mustard' – looking stuff. This is a sign your baby has passed all that meconium, which is good. If you don't notice this change by day five call your midwife for advice, just because she may want to assess a few other things to make sure your baby is feeding well.

As your baby gets older, you'll notice the poo is yellower. It should stay soft or even a bit runny and for the first four weeks you should see at least two poos a day. Sometimes breastfed babies can go a couple of days without pooing or they may seem to poo all the time. Either can be normal but talk to your midwife about this so they can double-check everything else is well.

TIP: EASY NAPPY CHANGING

When changing your baby's nappy (see also page 302), roll or fold up the dirty nappy under your baby first, clean your baby then pick him/her up onto one shoulder. Put the clean nappy down, open it up first then lay him/her on the nappy, rather than try to slide the nappy under your baby.

KEY POINTS

- Newborn skin is unique and goes through a highly sophisticated process after birth – cosmetic products cannot replace or become part of this process.
- It takes your baby at least four weeks to develop their own delicate protective barrier. Washing with soap can disrupt this natural process and hinder the skin's ability to do its job properly, so experts around the globe advise you only use water during this time.
- No wash products should be marketed as 'safe for newborns'.

Debrief before discharge

WHATEVER TYPE OF birth or wherever you gave birth, you will have some sort of birth debrief. A debrief gives you an opportunity to think or talk openly and honestly about your experience of birth. It is important that your story is acknowledged, even if that is only by you. Going through a debrief can help you make sense of what happened at the birth of your baby but also the deep emotions and feelings that went with it. Ideally you should have a debrief before you are discharged from your midwife by around day 10. There are a few different ways to debrief so this section will cover your options and how to go about debriefing.

THREE WAYS TO DEBRIEF

As you know, giving birth to another human is a huge deal. No matter what kind of birth or experience you had, try to record it before day 10 as every passing day with your baby is full of new memories you will probably forget things or they gradually become patchy.

1. **Write down your story:** Writing out your birth story helps to clear space and create room from any internal self-chatter you may have. Your birth story doesn't need to be particularly long or over-descriptive, just whatever works for you. Use writing as an outlet. As you run through it, write out any questions you have or anything that doesn't make sense. Time passes quickly in labour and your perception can become obscured so always write your take on what happened. Then, if you are happy with everything, it all adds up and makes sense, you don't need to do much

else other than add to it as and when you feel the need to. Some women end up turning this into a little diary log on their phone, with recordings and pictures to go with their journey into motherhood.

2. **Go through questions with a midwife:** If you have any questions or anything doesn't make sense, it's important to go through this with your midwife. Even if you can't see the midwife who looked after you in labour, a midwife will understand all of the medical terminology documented in your notes and be able to explain it to you. Whether it was a positive or difficult experience you need to know what happened, when and why. You might be given that tiny bit of information that then completes a whole puzzle in your head. It's a good idea to let your midwife know beforehand that you have a few questions and may need a little longer at your discharge appointment. If you need any follow-up care or appointments, your midwife can identify these and either signpost or make them for you.

3. **Birth reflections/debrief at hospital:** If your midwife can't answer all your questions, fill in certain gaps or you are struggling to come to terms with your birth experience, you may need to refer to the birth reflections or debrief service in your hospital. Don't feel silly asking for this; perhaps 80 per cent of your birth was perfect, but you have a niggling 20 per cent of doubt about what happened. All NHS maternity units offer some sort of service for postnatal women to discuss their care if they feel the need to. If you are having trouble accessing this you can email the Trust you received care from and request to see the birth reflections midwife or simply ask for a debrief. Bring your written questions with you to any follow-up appointments so you can get all the answers you need; you might be tired or go blank when you think about what you wanted to ask, so go prepared. Remember that this service exists to help you so ask and go through whatever it is you feel you need to.

SUNDAY BIRTH STORIES

There's such huge variation between what it means, looks and feels like to be a mother. As a midwife I am lucky enough to meet many mothers and to experience many births, whether a home birth, water birth, C-section, quick birth or pro-longed labour. But most people's version of birth is what they see in films and on TV – which as we know, is not a true reflection of birth. Rather than keep moaning about the media's version of birth I thought I'd try to help change it in some small way. I started a feature on Instagram called 'Sunday Birth Stories' where women send me their birth stories and I share them on my own Instagram story. I share as many different stories as possible from women all over the world. Pregnant women want and need to know about birth, and postnatal women want and need to share their birth story. There's no scaremongering, just good advice – remember Ina May Gaskins wise words, 'It's bad manners to scare pregnant women.'

When women send me their story, if something seems to be in the wrong order or they aren't clear on something, I ask if that is exactly what happened. I never suggest it is not, but just ask the question. Doing this with hundreds of women has taught me that sometimes memory jumps and misses sections or naturally forgets key points. Birth is such a profound experience that things can get hazy. Our memories influence how we think and feel about every aspect of our lives. In relation to birth; it is so important that you have an accurate memory of your birth: what happened, why and how. The best part about doing this feature is the feedback from women who send me their stories. Many say that writing it out really helped them understand and remember their birth.

I get daily messages from first-time mums explaining that seeing other women's births really helped them understand the different aspects of birth and what to potentially expect so they felt better prepared when they went into labour. They can see what a home birth looks like and what a C-section can look like and the realness of the post-baby body.

'I love the variety of birth experiences you share and it's so important for women to know that there are so many ways it can go. Luckily for me, everything worked out the way I hoped it would. But had it not, I would have known it was okay because of seeing other women's experiences.'

Emily, first-time mum

Many women have been so brave in sharing their intimate experiences and are very honest about how they felt and what they thought. This honesty leads to other mums feeling more normal about themselves and their situation. Knowing someone else feels or felt like you is like a weight being lifted. Writing out your birth story helps process your emotions and saves some details that may otherwise be forgotten.

As soon as I tell people that I am a midwife, some instantly start telling me their own experience of birth. It can be almost like they have been waiting to ask questions and get some answers from someone who might know. Women I have met for the first time can go into detail about their birth and how they felt. Sometimes at parties or weddings I have spent hours talking to women about their births because they have never got the explanation they needed to understand their own birth story.

Unfortunately, I can rarely give them all the answers they need as I don't have access to their medical notes, but just telling someone seems to really help. Many of these women have not had bad experiences either; they just haven't had the opportunity to acknowledge their own birth story properly. Doing the Sunday Birth Stories and talking to women as I have done over the years has taught me that most women need some sort of birth debrief and enjoy sharing their birth story.

'The following months were a conflict of sheer joy that he was here but also devastation at the way the birth had turned out. I had a crash C-section under a general anaesthetic because it was an emergency and it's very rare for this to happen. I went through every emotion of anger, sadness, jealousy and feeling guilty that I "shouldn't" feel this way because I had a healthy baby. I had some counselling to deal with this and learnt that it is perfectly okay and valid to feel conflicting emotions. It's valid to grieve for a missed birth and the things associated with that. They are independent events and having a healthy baby does not cancel out these feelings. It is so important for all mums to understand their birth story.'

Katie, first-time mum

WHEN DEBRIEFING MIGHT NOT BE FOR YOU

There is some evidence that shows there is no benefit in a debrief for women who have had traumatic experiences of birth, and that going through what happened with the notes may cause more trauma. Everyone experiences trauma differently, so if you are crying often about your birth, having nightmares or flashbacks, and often feeling anxious, it's important to address this as soon as possible with more specialist services, and your midwife, GP or health visitor can help you to access these. Evidence shows that the most crucial time to be seen is within the first month of a difficult or traumatic birth.

'I had a debrief at six weeks as I needed to know what happened and I'd definitely have another before or during another pregnancy. It was SO useful in helping to understand why Charles got stuck and to be able to express our point of view and where we felt things could have been more positive. As part of my debrief the visit to theatres was AMAZING; the consultant midwife took me around one quiet Sunday and we walked calmly from the labour ward to theatre, which last time had been running and terrifying. I saw where he was born and they explained what had happened in terms of resuscitation etc. It ended in the recovery room which I do remember so that was good. The experience felt like closure.'

Katie, first-time mum

Make Birth Better is a great campaign and their site has a really helpful map of local birth trauma support services so you can find out what's available to you in your area. Another brilliant support network full of information is Birth Trauma Association.

KEY POINTS

- We need to create a bigger and more realistic perspective of birth.
- Looking at different birth stories may help your perception of birth.
- One of the biggest stories story you'll ever tell is your birth story, so it's important to write it out.
- In any birth, understanding your experience is part of your recovery. Your birth experience seriously matters – you need to take time to process your emotions surrounding it.
- Ask anything and everything you need to about your birth.

Your new 'normal' and recognising problems

EVERYONE IS DIFFERENT and the boundaries of 'normality' are ever-changing according to culture and society. How you go about accepting your personal new normal may well be different to how your friend does it. As a new mum, drawing the line between what is normal to feel and experience and what is crossing over into illness can be hard.

Baby blues, postnatal depression (PND), anxiety and maternal mental health are topics that I could easily write an entire book about. Mental health illnesses are huge topics that we understand more about every day.

Often, it is the person closest to you who spots things early on and helps you recognise any concerns, so this is a good section for your partner to read too. Lots of women over the years have 'got on with it', marching on, wearing a Superwoman cape. Try to make a decision now to avoid this approach to the postnatal period, and your perception of depression, because 'marching on' often isn't sustainable.

Always talk to your midwife or GP if you have any concerns about your mental health.

ANXIETY, BABY BLUES AND DEPRESSION

Anxiety and depression are the most common mental health problems during pregnancy and after birth, and according to the NHS they affect around 10–

15 per cent of women. However, several cases go unreported, so I suspect that statistic merely scratches the surface. We know today that women are more likely to get PND if they have previously experienced mental health issues, have a lack of or a poor support system, or relationship difficulties. Previous abuse can also be a trigger. These are all factors to be aware of but at the same time suffering from a mental health illness can happen to anyone at any time.

Anxiety

Every day I meet mothers who experience anxiety about something, especially in those early weeks after a baby is born. Anxiety can come in the form of intrusive thoughts and some of these can be quite distressing. Mums don't often talk about intrusive thoughts and this can give them more power than they really deserve. For example, you may play out a scenario in your head that you would never do in real life, then you feel awful about thinking that and judge yourself. Most of us get intrusive thoughts and pass them off as ridiculousness but when you're a new mum you can start to judge yourself. Having negative thoughts does not make you a bad person or a bad mother. Your thoughts *don't* define you. Having said that, thoughts of self-harm or harming your baby are different. If you do get violent or aggressive thoughts you need to seek help urgently and don't be afraid of doing this.

Thoughts like, 'what if my baby becomes unwell ...' create fear and lack of confidence that you'll be able to deal with a situation you might be presented with. This then spirals off into unhelpful and negative ways of thinking about yourself. Generally, that is where anxiety stems from for new mums – they think they won't be able to deal with things they might be presented with.

You can manage and you will do just fine.

Pay attention to what you are worried about; look it in the face and question: what exactly am I worried about? Address the anxiety like you did with any fears around birth (see page 73) rather than let it spiral or beat yourself up about it. You might not love every new minute of motherhood and that's perfectly okay; it is hard work at times.

It's good to get comfortable with the fact you probably won't get to a place where you never worry about anything. Within reason, a certain amount of worrying serves a purpose: it's a defence mechanism and helps warn and prepare us. But, if it takes up too much of your time, stops you from doing things you want to do, and affects your quality of life, then the balance has been tipped from useful to harmful. If that's the case, it's important to seek help for your anxiety so you can manage it properly.

It can be helpful to learn strategies to calm your body down. I'm a fan of body scanning, where you pay attention to the parts of your body that are changing when you feel anxious. For example, anxiety may make you feel sick, increase your heart rate, or make you sweat. Scan your body from head to toe, drop your shoulders, relax and breathe deeply into each part of your body. This can help to relieve the feelings of anxiety. It can also help to run through the following five thoughts:

1. Is this thought useful?
2. Remember, you are not your thoughts.
3. The only thing you can really control is yourself.
4. Drop your shoulders, create space for yourself and breathe deep.
5. Surrender to the present moment – it is what it is.

Being prepared in practical ways can help your mindset too. One woman I saw told me about one of the first times she went out with her newborn, she forgot an umbrella and it rained. But the next time she remembered and she happened to have an appointment with me. The first thing she said was 'look' holding the umbrella like a baton, 'I've got my shit together today. I've got my umbrella!' As silly as it may sound, it is important to give yourself credit for what appear to be small things in motherhood – if you get out of the house with everything you need and arrive somewhere on time – winning! Celebrate the small successes, because you've got a big job and you're doing great.

'Difficult roads often lead to beautiful destinations'

– MELCHOR LIM

Baby blues

There's a difference between 'baby blues' and postnatal Depression (PND). Baby blues affect at least 60 per cent, perhaps even up to 80 per cent of women in the postnatal period. It usually kicks in around three to five days after having a baby. It is due to the fluctuation of hormones, lack of sleep, the mind-blowing event of giving birth, any postnatal pain you are having to deal with, and the fact you have just become a mother. Baby blues are waves of emotions combined with a cocktail of hormones resulting in a tearful period. It can leave some women feeling low or anxious for a few days, and it is also common to over-react to things. Go easy on yourself. It's okay to cry and get irritable. It's just a natural phase, just like the transition in labour and the birth pause (see page 224). Like those two phases you may have already experienced, this too will come and then go. Be prepared to feel like this and let it all out.

'The first two weeks were the hardest; I felt sick from all the meds so the smell of Charles's milk made me feel sick. I was in a lot of pain from a wound infection and wanted to run away every day, but felt this huge sense of responsibility because "the mum can never run". I wrote a list that I would add to every time I thought of something of all the things I knew I wanted to do with Charles (beach visits, farm visits, etc.) It gave me something to look forward to and focus on the future when I knew I would be pain-free and feel better mentally. Seven months later I am more connected to my baby than ever, he is my little mate, he reaches for me when he is tired and he has a special smile that only I seem to get. I didn't see him born but that becomes less and less relevant as each day passes; I was the cause of his first smile, I have seen his first roll, I fed him his first food, and I'll be there for all his other firsts. There is no greater truth than "time is the best healer".'

Kate, first-time mum

Postnatal depression

Women often feel guilty or scared to admit they have PND, especially as they were expecting to be happy about having a baby and everyone around them was expecting the same. All of these perceptions and feelings about PND are common but these feelings can delay recovery because admitting there is a problem is the first step to recovery. The more we all talk about PND, the more we all learn, so it can become less a condition to feel embarrassed about, and more something that we can ask for support for. It breaks my heart when I hear women say, 'Maybe it's just me, I'm not good enough. I can't cope.' Please don't ever feel like it is just you who feels like this, it's not. You are good enough. PND is an illness and not something that makes you a bad or weak mum.

The symptoms of PND are similar to those in depression at other times, and include prolonged low mood, feeling irritable, exhausted and not getting pleasure from things you normally would. It can start in late pregnancy, after the birth or start later on. It really does vary in severity and timing. One woman said to me, 'My husband knew something was seriously up when I shovelled my favourite burger into my mouth without any sign of pleasure, noises of "mmmm" or comments. I'm not joking, that was what led to my diagnosis.' This new mum couldn't see it herself but the lack of enjoyment was genuinely the final clue for her partner. He thought she was down but when she gained no pleasure from something she always loved – he knew he needed to help her get better.

There is no physical test for PND, and interestingly, psychiatry is one of the only specialities that doesn't always look at what they need to treat first. If someone has a stroke, they will have brain scans and MRIs, but when it comes to diagnosing and treating mental illness it's rare that we look at the structure of the brain first, although some neuroscientists and psychiatrists are starting to do this pre-diagnosis.

As a rough guideline, if you find symptoms are persisting for more than two weeks then you need to seek help from your doctor. They will run through some questions to diagnose PND and then offer help, perhaps therapy or medication. If you are diagnosed with PND it's important to remember you are not letting anyone down. Speaking to your doctor will mark the beginning of your journey towards feeling better. Depending on your specific symptoms, your doctor will work with you to make a plan. Sometimes the doctor may prescribe medication and it is very common to worry about the effect that the pills may have on your baby if you are breastfeeding. Rest assured that the doctor would not prescribe anything to you that could harm your baby, and the most important thing for the health of your baby is to have a healthy mother.

'I had expected motherhood to be this wonderful thing, but it wasn't. I just didn't feel attached to her, with my feelings going from just wanting to leave the house to wanting to go back to work and my normal life! Sisterhood is such an important support network that I was craving. All I wanted was my mum to come and take care of me and guide me through. My husband was very supportive during this time, but it was my mum who I needed. She'd had four children and breastfed us all for over a year; it was her experience I wanted. The turning point for me was my health visitor who was just great, I was really open and honest and expressed my concerns about PND and she arranged a follow-up a week later. After my follow-up and once we got past the first two weeks, I felt completely different and had started to turn a corner. I have since found some excellent profiles online which are just honest about things. I wished I'd had these in my early days when I worried it was just me who felt lonely, out of my depth and overwhelmed with this huge life change.'

Ellie, midwife and first-time mum

One thing worth mentioning here is that if you have been given medication, and a few months have passed and you are feeling better, you should speak to your doctor about whether or not to continue with it. You should have been given this advice from the beginning but might not have taken it in at the time. Generally, this type of medication will be given alongside talking therapy of some sort, so it is also worth visiting your doctor every once in a while to give an update on how that is going so that your records are up to date and that everyone has the full picture.

POSTNATAL DEPRESSION AND PARTNERS

It is not only mums who suffer from mental health problems in the postnatal period; it is thought that between 4–25 per cent of men have PND in the two months following birth. The onset can be more gradual than it is in women. Dads can often feel lonely and disconnected from their friends, especially if they are caring for a mum who has PND. One factor is that men tend to talk less about it. Women are sometimes a bit better at coming forward and admitting that there is a problem, while men can suffer in silence. A campaign that I have seen on social media recently nailed it with one question: #howareyoudad. It is important to keep asking your partner how they are too.

It is difficult sometimes amidst all the nappies, feeding and lack of sleep to take care of one another like you used to and to really notice how the other one is feeling. The baby comes first and that is completely natural. A friend of mine and her partner decided to set an alarm on their phones for every five days at the same time, and they dedicated ten minutes to just being open about how they were feeling that week. If they couldn't do it right away, they would snooze the alarm until they could. It started as a joke to begin with, but once they got into the habit it became something that they both started to depend on. Their baby is now three years old and they still have a regular catch-up out of habit.

If you notice that something doesn't seem quite right, then have a chat with your partner even if the baby is crying in the background and it's short and sweet. Then set aside some time to make a plan together to seek help. It sometimes helps to remind one another that you are not just parents, but partners too, and that you are in this together.

If you want to know more about PND, www.rcpsych.ac.uk have a lot of up-to-date information. There are also charities such as PANDAS Foundation and Cocoon Family Support that you can call and get support from. These charities are open to anyone, and offer peer support, walking groups and courses.

MYTH: I HAD THE PERFECT BIRTH SO I WON'T GET PND

Postnatal depression is not dependent on the type of birth that you have. Sometimes there is an assumption that a woman who has had a straightforward birth that went according to plan will, and should be, mentally well. That is not the case, and it's not for us to diagnose 'mental health' based on birth experience. A difficult or traumatic birth is more likely to impact mental health, but that doesn't mean to say if you have had a positive birth experience you won't get baby blues or postnatal depression. Please don't feel unworthy of seeking help after your dream birth. The change of identity and shift into motherhood can be destabilising for everyone.

WHO AM I?

You might not feel depressed but you just might not feel like yourself. One day in your postpartum period you may walk past a mirror and not recognise your own reflection and one day you may ask yourself, 'Who am I?' It's normal. Almost every first-time mum I have looked after goes through some sort of identity crisis. Some are very minor fleeting thoughts and some are intensely confusing. Research shows that on average it takes *two to four years* for women to feel like 'themselves' again after having a baby (just about the time you might be thinking of having another one!). If you have been used to working set hours, with a busy independent routine, it may take time to accept the changes you are now facing. Even when you go back to work and 'normal life' you may not really feel like yourself for a long time. Try not to judge who you have become: you're a strong woman and someone's mum. You're doing so well managing everything. Be mindful of the way you are talking to yourself; sometimes the things we say to ourselves are shocking and if another person said those things we may call it domestic abuse. We have learned to be harsh on ourselves; as children, when we look in the mirror we are wowed, intrigued and beautiful – it is only as we get older we start to compare and judge ourselves. Try to talk to yourself the way you would talk to a close friend who you love and care about.

In any major life change there is a loss, even the changes you're truly grateful for. There is a sort of grief that comes with this loss, but in new motherhood the feeling of grief coexists with joy and shows you a whole new level of strength you never knew you had.

'I really struggled the first month after having Luca. You know you are going to have a baby but NOTHING can prepare you for how little time you have to yourself. After a C-section I had to take things even easier than a vaginal labour. My normal way of being "Nadz" would be going to a gym class, getting my nails done or my eyebrows. During pregnancy, I was still doing all that so it was a massive change, let alone having a baby to look after as well.

'A big part of my life before becoming a mum was my routine and that goes out of the window with a baby so you have all of these emotions and frustration because you are literally in the great unknown. Someone said to me it's important to still have "you time", even if you have a baby. My immediate reaction was "Oh God, how selfish." But it wasn't until I accepted that and got my mum to come over and I went to dye my hair (only upstairs mind, but still) that I started to slowly but surely feel like me again.'

Nadz, first-time mum

A good analogy that I tell women about, is the temperature of the shower. A hot shower is unpleasant and so is a cold shower, but when you mix the two it's lovely, it can just take a little adjusting to get the temperature that's right for you. This is a fine balance that is slightly different for everyone too. I may find your shower too hot. So, try not to focus on what works for other mums if it simply isn't working for you. Having a rule early on of taking just a few minutes a day to yourself is the best way to avoid getting lost in nappies.

'Take ten minutes time out away from the baby every day, from newborn. Even just ten minutes of breathing and listening to fave music in another room, a bath, really enjoying a hot cup of tea, or walk outside without the baby. This saved me and reminded me every day of who I was. Not just a mummy.'

Katie, mum of one and expecting baby number two

THE MIND–BODY CONNECTION

~~~~~

As I mentioned, PND can happen to anyone, but there are a few things you might find interesting about depression in general. There are some recent discoveries about depression and neuroimmunology, a field combining neuroscience, the study of the nervous system, and the immune system. More than 100 trillion bacteria are living and working in your gut and collectively these microorganisms are referred to as the microbiome. The microbiome is thought to help our body in a number of ways, like processing nutrients, digestion and producing immune molecules that heal wounds and fighting inflammation. A new theory is emerging that there is a stronger connection between our gut and brain than was originally thought. Dr Edward Bullmore has a brilliant book called *The Inflamed Mind* that gives more insight into the relationship between inflammation and depression. In short, and grossly simplified, he explains that inflammation has an effect on human behaviour. The inflammation proteins and cells in the body directly change the way our brains work, which in turn changes thoughts and behaviour.

The brain and immune function were believed to have nothing to do with each other. Some experts mistakenly thought the blood–brain barrier protected the brain from inflammation in the body, dividing the mind and body into two separate entities. We now know that cytokines (inflammation signallers) do in fact get through the blood–brain barrier, and pro-inflammatory cytokines increase in the third trimester of pregnancy. Bullmore explains that inflammation (see page 320) in the brain may have a link to depression – around 40 per cent of depressed patients are also inflamed. We used to think of depression as all about the mind but we need to think about how the body affects the brain too. What I like particularly about this latest science is that it helps us move away from stigma and self-criticism and towards understanding. The belief that inflammation in the body affects the brain's function means we should be able to talk more openly about our struggles rather than feel ashamed or become a victim of self-blame.

It's important to bear in mind that there could also be other underlying physical causes for PND, for example, an underactive thyroid or low levels of vitamin B. I have seen a few women diagnosed with hypothyroidism after years of believing they had depression all that time. The symptoms are very similar, so blood tests can be worth considering too.

INFLAMMATION IN THE BODY

Before we go into anti-inflammatory living, it is important to note that this theory is new and the word 'inflammation' is a bit of a buzz word. The evidence surrounding inflammation in the body and its potential effect on the mind is not entirely conclusive – the jury is still out. Being diagnosed with depression doesn't mean that you have inflammation and vice versa. Just to be clear, it is possible that having PND has nothing to do with inflammation. Having said that, the tips below lead to a healthier lifestyle anyway, and if science is able to prove a definitive link between inflammation and depression it is a win – win all round. Here are some things to think about, to reduce your chances of inflammation in the body:

- **Hydration.** Hydrating really well helps to keep things moving through the liver, kidneys and bowels. Generally speaking, the more hydrated you are, the less inflammation in your body. Aim for about 2–2.5 litres per day (see page 268). Chlorine isn't good for us or for the microbiome; if you haven't already then consider investing in a decent water filter for your tap water. They're not too expensive and well worth it. There's also the (more expensive option) of fitting a filter at source, under the kitchen tap – the water will also taste better.
- **Daily movement.** As Robyn mentioned on page 260, you're not going to be doing a HIIT workout soon after you have had a baby, but gentle daily movement is important. Daily movement can simply be walking around your garden or house or swaying on the spot with your baby. Massages also help get your circulation moving. You can gradually increase the intensity of your daily movement over time and many of the classes you did in pregnancy like yoga or Pilates will offer postnatal classes and advice too. It is recommended that you leave it at least three months before returning to running.
- **Meditation.** I can't emphasise the benefits of meditation enough. The world's leading scientists, philosophers and physicists now agree that meditation reduces anxiety and increases mental control and overall happiness by allowing the mind to find peace with the present moment. EEGs (Electroencephalogram) performed on monks highlighted a clear difference in brainwave activity. As a professional who is sceptical, interested in evidence and first-hand experiences, I went to a monastery in Tibet to find out more for myself. I spent 11 days with a female monk ten hours from the city I landed in. We slept in the same room and spent the best part of 24 hours a day together. I learnt so much about my mental health and I found true inner peace through meditation. It

can take a while to learn how to meditate, especially if you are feeling depressed, but there are classes you can attend or apps you can use to learn gradually.

- **Diet.** Nourish your brain with healthy fats such as avocado, eggs, olive oil, flaxseeds and nuts. Reducing the amount of refined carbs in your diet like white bread, pastries and biscuits is helpful. Grains are good to eat, along with probiotics like kimchi (fermented pickle) and kefir but you can take probiotic supplements if you prefer (see page 270). Turmeric has been ingested for years and is thought to have various benefits; I have it fresh every morning in hot water with black pepper and manuka honey (hot water and black pepper helps you absorb the nutrients from turmeric). Fruits like berries, lemons and limes are great for anti-inflammatory properties too. (See page 268 for more on postnatal nutrition.)

- **Stress.** When you feel stressed or overwhelmed the body goes into 'fight or flight' mode. The body thinks you need to run away or fight to save your life and in response hormones are released to help you do just that. When you are in fight or flight mode for an extended period of time your body is surviving not thriving. Inflammation in the body is a response to a threat, whether it's a foreign invader, like bacteria or virus, and even a psychological or emotional 'threat' that leads to stress. In response to this, the immune system sends out an army of molecules, called pro-inflammatory cytokines, to attack the invaders.

YOUR BEST SELF

At times, motherhood may feel like you've been given a challenge that is almost too hard for you. But being in that place is where humans can really grow and reach their higher self. Every new mum goes through some form of emotional struggle, and accepting your new normal can be a challenge in itself. Your energy, body and mind are focused on being a mother. The truth is your best self is all you can ever be. You are doing a great job. Forgive yourself for the tiny errors you make, try not to over think or question your own judgement, and remember to be kind to yourself.

KEY POINTS

- Seek support early on if you have any concerns over your mental health.
- The most common mental health illnesses after having a baby are anxiety and depression.
- Remember to check in with your partner too.
- The more open everyone is about mental illness the better our understanding will be.
- Things that are good for your body are also good for your mind.
- Self-care is simple and you need to dedicate time to it.
- Prevent and reduce inflammation.
- You can only ever be your best self.

It takes a village to raise a mum

THEY SAY IT takes a village to raise a child, but the same can be said for raising a mum. For the whole of human history we have mostly evolved to raise children in tribes and villages. Traditionally, women would learn from their own mums, sisters, cousins and other women in their villages; the elders in the village passed on their wisdom. Understanding birth, breastfeeding and all the changes motherhood brings was part of growing up, was learned behaviour and was openly talked about. In many places around the world this is how women learn about motherhood; the elders teach them. As we don't live like this any more in the Western world, we have a bit of a broken chain of wisdom. Rarely is the type of support you need as a new mum (especially in the postnatal period) talked about. In this section we will rebuild some links and find out why it takes a village to raise a mum and how to build your own modern-day village.

YOUR NEW COPING STRATEGIES

The chances are that at some point in your life you have felt a little 'out of sync' or unsure about yourself, and you found coping strategies to help, such as a night out, a few drinks, an evening run, reading a book, or watching a film (from start to finish). These things aren't so easy to do with a tiny baby. Having people to lean on helps you create new coping strategies for the various changes you're going through as a new mum.

When you start a new job, just knowing who you can go for lunch with gives you a feeling of safety and stability. This scenario is so similar to new motherhood; treat it as though you're going into a new work place with a brand-new role – you need to have that bit of stability and support from someone else. It is even better when it's someone else who has a little more experience than you. We have been sold the idea of independence and strength, which is great and I'm all for independent women, but that sometimes makes new mums feel like they shouldn't need anyone to lean on. There's no shame in needing a friend, so try to put yourself out there and make new friends whenever you can. It can change everything.

Asking for help

When it comes down to it, we're pretty bad at asking for help and sometimes even accepting help. Honestly, no one is going to think any less of you for reaching out. Imagine one of your good friends calling you right now and saying, 'I'm struggling a bit this week, could you pop round at some point? I'm so tired and just need a bit of help.' Would you think any less of her? Your close friends will understand if you reach out. Most people are happy to help if you ask and when help is offered, why say no?

Creating your own village can also mean moving away from people or things that are causing you more stress. Minimise contact with those who are unhelpful or overly critical. You may even need to cut them off if you feel it's necessary. As harsh as that sounds it can be liberating. Toxic, jealous or insecure people won't help you build and sustain your nest – they won't help to raise you. On the positive side, now might be a good time to move towards that joker you know. Everyone knows a joker and laughter is known to have similar effects to antidepressants because it raises serotonin levels. Laughter and not taking yourself so seriously won't cure a mental health problem, and I'd never mask the darkness of loneliness and depression with 'just laugh it off and you'll be fine' – but finding ways to enjoy yourself can help you deal with the more difficult days.

Meeting and hanging out with like-minded parents helps to normalise your transition and change of identity. You can bounce things off each other, laugh things off, run things by each other and most importantly not feel judged. Large-scale research over many years shows that with a good support network, parents can and do feel more confident in their role. Look up local support groups, mother and baby groups, mums' meet ups or digital networks like Channel Mum and apps like Lets Mush or Mums Anywhere.

'Three words ... FIND. YOUR. TRIBE! Join mums' groups, music groups, local toddler groups, libraries ... keep trying until you find the people who you click with and then mum date them!'

Jessica, second-time mum

MATRESCENCE

Alexandra Sacks has a TED Talk on the discovery of 'Matrescence', a word describing the transition from woman to mother. The main point she makes is about the fact that we all remember going through adolescence; we were hormonal, moody, sometimes confused, had break-outs and our bodies grew in strange places at fast paces, and at the same time people expected you to be grown up in a new way. When you think about it, adolescent changes are similar to the changes you go through as a new mum. Matrescence is the word she suggests we use to describe this transformation.

We know it's normal for teenagers to feel a bit unsure of themselves so she asks, 'Why don't we think about pregnancy and the postnatal period in the same way as adolescence?' Sacks points out that we have entire books written on the developmental and physical changes of adolescents, but we don't even have a word to describe the transition to motherhood. The changes motherhood bring can lead to an upheaval of emotions and questions about how you feel you fit into the world. By talking to others and being honest about how you feel, even to that mum who looks confident, you'll discover that most mums feel the same way.

Remember that your version of motherhood doesn't have to look like a way that makes other people feel comfortable. You should do what you want, when you want and how you want to. Challenging the expectations can be hard, but motherhood is liberating in that you can break away from any oppressive cultural norms and limitations. You can reinvent things and teach your baby what *you* want to.

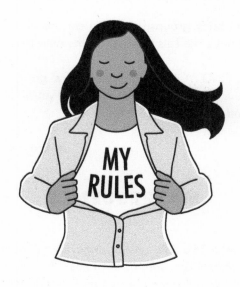

SHARING YOUR THOUGHTS

~~~~

When we spend a lot of time with babies, who, when young, are non-verbal creatures, we start to talk to ourselves, often internally. On average we have between 60,000–90,000 thoughts per day. If your partner goes back to work and you spend a lot of time alone with your baby, the chances are that some negative thoughts will start to creep in. Someone else needs to hear these thoughts in order for you to physically get rid of them. Having a get-together morning once a week with other parents is really beneficial for your mental health – research shows that a good social network could actually extend your life expectancy. If there's no local groups on regularly enough for you, organise your own mumma morning. Ask all the mums you know, your friends of friends, brother's girlfriend's friends with babies ... and any other mums that live nearby. Good relationships and social lives are so good for human health.

Social interaction activates the genes in your body that help your immune system fight against diseases. The University of California did a study and found that women with breast cancer are *four times* more likely to recover successfully if they have a strong connection with a supportive group of friends and family. The power of connecting with someone and being honest changes the brain's chemistry. We get a flood of two happy hormones, dopamine and oxytocin – these hormones can help you cope better with the tougher days and the sleep deprivation that new mumhood brings.

Life won't be like it was before baby arrived, but once you create your own modern village you will have deep and very meaningful, honest and frank relationships that can enhance your life.

KEY POINTS

- There's no shame in needing a friend; do put yourself out there.
- Ask for help if and when you need it.
- Matrescence is like adolescence.
- Social interaction changes brain chemistry.
- Your mum mates are some of the best mates you'll make.

How to live in the digital age as a new mum

WE ARE LIVING in such a unique time, some historians and philosophers have labelled it a 'digital revolution'. We have a world of information constantly at our fingertips, and there's not much you can't find out within seconds online. As well as having access to an overwhelming amount of information, we also have insight into everyone else's life. Can you remember what it was like trying to keep in contact with all your friends before social media? Or having to wait for songs to come on the radio to hear them? We have seen and been through the progression of the digital age, but our babies will be the first generation in human history to grow up with ask Alexa, take a ride in a driverless car and have their lives digitally documented.

The digital age is progressing at such a fast pace and is clearly here to stay. It is important that you use what is available wisely, like connecting with other parents (see page 135 on meet-up apps) yet also give some thought to how to manage the side of the digital age that can be unhelpful.

DIGITAL ADDICTION?

Online content has become part of what's known as the 'attention economy' due to our ever-increasing focus on smartphones. A *Time* magazine poll found that 84 per cent of people are attached to their phones on a daily basis, with 20 per cent checking them every 10 minutes, and these stats are in line with other findings in relation to smartphone usage.

Part of the attraction to smartphones comes from the rush of endorphins (happy hormones) they deliver. Scientists have found that every time we receive a notification of a like, share, retweet or comment, the pleasure centre of our brain receives a satisfying rush of these neurochemicals. Simon Sinek, TED speaker, the author of multiple bestselling books and social-media influencer, talks about the dangers of digital addiction and he goes as far as saying that social media has the same effect on the brain as some drugs, alcohol and gambling – yet there are no regulations for it. He is most concerned about children and teenagers and their increasingly high dependence to be 'liked' or 'followed' online.

Our brains have developed to operate in a certain way as part of evolution. We're hard-wired to get distracted, stop, assess and analyse things, so no matter how hard we try, sometimes switching off or disengaging with your digital device is hard to do.

A 2009 study of macaque monkeys showed that when primates receive information, their dopamine systems are activated too, just like when they find food. If we apply that to humans it may explain why we end up having our phone in one hand, the TV on and the Kindle on the side table. The hit of happy hormones that come from likes and receiving new information actually feels good.

Our human 'need to know' mentality also makes navigating new motherhood even harder. We all want the best for our babies and there are also physiological rewards that feel good from gaining information. By combing those two desires you're particularly vulnerable to the downfall of the digital age and information overload. Not to mention the fact that most apps and websites are specifically designed to grab our attention and keep us exploring them. Social media platforms allow people to see you're 'active' or have seen their message, making us feel obliged to reply. Many women tell me about how they end up in a social-media 'hole' after opening the app first thing when on maternity leave. Before they know it they've lost half an hour scrolling, liking, following, watching, shopping and the list goes on. The brain is so well stimulated and satisfied on social media it is difficult to get off, out and meet people in 'the real world'. You can feel connections from people online but as we will go on to talk about – nothing beats physical communication, seeing people's faces and getting a hug. Far less of your senses and human needs are met through a screen.

THE POSITIVES

Most of us use some form of social-media platform and overall social media has a lot of power. Research shows that social-media users generally fall into one of two categories: 'Meformers', who make up about 80 per cent of users, and mostly post information about themselves, and 'Informers', who make up about 20 per cent of users, and post information that isn't immediately related to themselves.

Regardless of what category they fall into, social media has given some people a voice who wouldn't traditionally have had a voice and platform to influence thousands of other people. In some way I believe it has given traditional mass media less power because the general public can share things, publicly challenge journalism and politics, and openly speak up against things or protest to drive change. Another area that has a lot of online positives are TED Talks, podcasts health apps or YouTubers offering educational or motivational talks and support.

There is a whole new world of celebrities made online who have been chosen by the public as opposed to by the press. I have built a communications platform with both women and midwives on social media. I'm grateful to be living in this time and to have the opportunity to spread messages and communicate so easily with women from all over the world. The simple fact is there is no way I would have had the impact I have had so far without social media.

Aside from giving people a voice, spreading messages and driving change, it's a great way to stay in contact with friends who don't live near you as they can catch up on your life and stay close to what's going on with you.

Some social-media accounts are just brilliant for new and expectant mums because they help to educate women about what to expect and give insight into what's normal. As I've mentioned (see page 172), if you're on social media, follow positive accounts to create your own narrative and understanding of motherhood. Lots of women I meet also build their tribes off the back of social media and have their own groups or look to forums for help and support. The internet is a great place to search and find events and groups in your local area. Messaging your WhatsApp group at 4am and getting an instant response can help you feel less alone as the rest of the world sleeps soundly.

We are lucky to reap the benefits that social media and digital access bring but, like most good things, it has its downside, and some of those can be particularly damaging to new mums. A bit more on this now.

THROUGH THE EYES OF THE FILTER

Social media is rarely an accurate reflection of real life. For some it's simply a well-planned business and for others it's a way to portray their life in its best form. Many people only post about the good times (#blessed) and rarely document the bad times. We are literally looking at people's lives through a filter. We've all seen contradicting posts people put out there and you can probably think of someone now who couldn't be further from what they portray themselves as on social media. You need to protect yourself in early motherhood, because you're perhaps more sensitive, self-critical and doubtful than usual, so the images of perfect families and postnatal bodies could make you doubt yourself and even resent your own reflection. Photos can be easily edited, Photoshopped, touched up to create illusions. Make a conscious decision to remember this when seeing a new mum with a flat tum; managing your social media influences at this time in your life is a must.

Being behind a screen changes people's behaviour too. Most of us will have read comments or responses and thought, I wonder if you would say *that* to their face? Keyboard warriors are a phenomenon that psychologists refer to as 'toxic disinhibition'. This is the idea that because the recipient of the message isn't physically tangible, an individual is more likely to make online statements that they wouldn't face-to-face. Online bullying and trolling are a big problem because people can hide behind a device or perhaps even a fake account. These keyboard warriors can cause serious anxiety, and comments on your personal life can really hurt at any time but especially when you're feeling a bit vulnerable in Matrescence.

CONSUMPTION AND STAYING HEALTHY

There is a natural tendency for humans to seek out information that confirms our own opinions ('confirmation bias'). We tend, therefore, to follow people on social media who reflect that. You may have created a digital world that suits your own bias. It's so easily done and I think we're all guilty of it at times in some shape or form; simply being aware of the narrative that serves your own bias is healthy and well-balanced.

I hear quite a lot about how new mothers feel obliged to answer messages and can be inundated and overwhelmed, just when they don't need it. It's often just well-wishers, relatives who are eager to get news and people wanting updates. But as a result of living in the digital age, what we've all come to expect are answers now. We know that we have control of our devices and can turn them off whenever we like, but those of us who are used to being on their phones a lot may find this difficult. If you can't bring yourself to switch it off totally you can always go into your settings and turn off notifications that pop up and disrupt your peace. Choose a time when you feel able to deal with messages – like when you are in a bit more of a routine and know your baby will be napping around 11am, or even set up an automatic response to say you can't reply at the moment. You can also unsubscribe from companies that fill your email inbox with *their* marketing material, adding little value to *your* life or direct more messages to your spam folder.

To help manage your digital exposure, consider unsubscribing yourself from everything that's not useful at this time, only keeping a small number of blogs, apps and podcasts that add value to your life as a new mum. There's an increasing demand for services like Unroll Me which can help you do this quickly or the app RescueTime. Facebook newsfeed eradicator can help you avoid the distractions of the internet for longer periods of time. Stay connected to the digital world, but only in a way that suits you.

Try to take digital breaks too ('digital detox' is becoming trendy); having a little time away from technology may give you more time for your own mental space and peace. I used to live on Instagram and decided to set myself some rules. I don't open Instagram until midday on Tuesday and Friday mornings, and as sad as it sounds, that time away has had a massive impact on my mornings. I feel far more in tune with myself and have a chance to think about me before I open up to what's going on in the rest of the world or respond to other people's requests. Setting this rule is a form of self-care; what other people are doing or want from you is not as important as what you are doing and what you need from yourself.

Another good tip is to avoid posting for the approval of a hypothetical audience in your head. Instead, try to create for yourself, your family and for the joy that comes from the creative and adaptive process of motherhood. There is a current movement of parents who are choosing not to post any photos of their children on social media without their consent. Instead, they have their own private album of photos on their phone/digital device or a WhatsApp group with their family for sharing cute snaps.

GOING OLD-SCHOOL

You probably have an old-school photo album somewhere that your mum/dad/nan created but because your baby is living in the digital age, you'll have so many memories you can easily capture for them. We live in a slightly different time, where the cameras are better quality and therefore a little less forgiving. However, one day your baby will treasure these digital memories so no matter how big you feel, what your hair looks like, or whether or not you've had a shower, your (grown-up) baby will want to see your face. So take lots of photos that include you!

Get in all the photos and videos because if you dig out those old-school photo albums I bet you don't look at one photo and think, 'Mum looks awful, don't think she showered that day.' You're more intrigued and grateful to see her younger self.

SCREEN TIME AROUND YOUR BABY

~

Lastly, there is a theory that when parents use technology frequently and for extended periods of time it can have negative effects on their child's development. Babies need a lot of sensory interaction so they can mimic and learn about the world and universal laws. Mirroring is when they observe and copy you, in everything that you do. This impacts how they develop socially and intellectually. When you're reading a post on social media or texting, your face is usually fairly emotionless – like it is as you're reading this now. Research has shown that emotionless expressions can be distressing for babies, especially when they are trying to engage with their parents. When you are fully engaged you show your baby a wide range of facial expressions, language and sounds. The brain of a young baby is shaped by the interactions they have with their parents and familiar people, and as mentioned this starts at a very early age (see page 282). It not realistic or necessary to completely stop using your phone and other devices around your baby, but it's important to be aware of your use.

KEY POINTS

- We are living in the digital age for the first time in human history.
- The digital age has given people a platform to help new mums connect with each other.
- We get a rush of happy hormones from likes but nothing beats face-to-face interaction.
- You control your devices, so unsubscribe and pay attention only to what matters in your life.
- Capturing new mum moments are so precious, and that includes yourself.
- Remember that your expressions really matter to your baby and if you're on your devices a lot you'll be less expressive.

A final note

I am a little sad we've got to the end now; writing this book has reminded me once again how amazing us women and our bodies are.

More than anything, I hope you feel more confident about your abilities and now have a few more tools to navigate your pregnancy, to make decisions, to manage your birth and early motherhood, and feel good about this transformative journey you are on.

What an incredible time it is to be a mother.

Motherhood shows you that you have a whole other level of strength you never knew you had. Remember, all you can ever do is your best, which is more than enough.

You have so got this.

Love

Marie Louise x

Helpful resources

GENERAL INFORMATION AND EVIDENCE

NHS www.nhs.uk/conditions/pregnancy-and-baby/

Cochrane www.cochrane.org

National Institute for Clinical Excellence www.nice.org.uk

RCOG www.rcog.org.uk

Department of Health (DOH) www.gov.uk/government/organisations/department-of-health-and-social-care

World Health Organisation (WHO) www.who.int

Nursing and Midwifery Council www.nmc.org.uk

Sarah Wickham www.sarawickham.com

Katie Hinde mammalssuck.blogspot.com

British Medical Journal (BMJ) journals.bmj.com/

Tommys Charity www.tommys.org

AIMS www.aims.org.uk

Maternity Transformation Programme www.england.nhs.uk/mat-transformation/prog-board

Antenatal classes
Better births www.betterbirthsanc.com

Yoga bellies www.yogabellies.co.uk

Active birth www.activebirthcentre.com

NCT nct.org.uk

Optimal fetal positioning
Spinning Babies spinningbabies.com

Active Birth www.janetbalaskas.com

Birth
Birth rights www.birthrights.org.uk

Positive birth movement www.positivebirthmovement.org

Doula UK doula.org.uk

Independent Midwives imuk.org.uk

Make Birth Better www.makebirthbetter.org

Birth Trauma Association birthtraumaassociation.org.uk

Better Births Campaign www.england.nhs.uk/wp-content/uploads/2016/02/national-maternity-review-report.pdf

Health
The Pregnancy Food Company www.thepregnancyfoodcompany.co.uk

Baby Safe Paint www.little-knights.co.uk

Shoppers Guide to Pesticides www.ewg.org/foodnews/clean-fifteen.php

Diabetes UK www.diabetes.org.uk

Screening tests
Government website www.gov.uk/government/publications/screening-tests-for-you-and-your-baby

Sleep
Precious Little Sleep www.preciouslittlesleep.com

Helping your baby to sleep: Your pregnancy and baby guide www.nhs.uk/conditions/pregnancy-and-baby/getting-baby-to-sleep

Lullaby Trust www.lullabytrust.org.uk/safer-sleep-advice

Infant feeding and bonding

UNICEF Baby Friendly Initiative www.babyfriendly.org.uk

La Leche League www.laleche.org.uk; Breastfeeding Helpline 0345 120 2918

Association of Breastfeeding Mothers abm.me.uk

Human Milk for Human Babies Facebook groups

Mental health

Perinatal Positivity perinatalpositivity.org

Best Beginnings www.bestbeginnings.org.uk/out-of-the-blue

Action on Post Partum Psychosis app-network.org

Tommy's charity www.tommys.org/pregnancy-information/im-pregnant/mental-health-during-and-after-pregnancy

Panda Foundation www.pandasfoundation.org.uk

Cocoon Family Support cocoonfamilysupport.org

Car seats

www.childcarseats.org.uk

Domestic Abuse Help

REACH 0800 088 4194

National Domestic Abuse Helpline 0808 2000247

Maternity Leave

www.gov.uk/maternity-pay-leave/leave

Maternity Action maternityaction.org.uk

Recommended TED Talks

Ina May Gaskin 'Reducing fear of birth in US culture'

Jill Bolte Taylor 'My stroke of insight'

Karni Liddell 'A happy baby'

Debrah Lewis 'Why fathers should be present at birth'

Katie Hinde 'What we don't know about mother's milk'

Penelope Jagessar Chaffer 'The toxic baby'

Alexandra Sacks 'Matrescence'

References

Sandall J, Soltani H, Gates S, Shennan A, Devane D www.cochrane.org/CD004667/PREG_midwife-led-continuity-models-care-compared-other-models-care-women-during-pregnancy-birth-and-earl (28 April 2016)

Healthy Baby Cohort study 'Afternoon napping during pregnancy and low birth weight: the Healthy Baby Cohort study', Song L, Shen L, Li H, Liu B, Zheng X, Zhang L, Xu S, Wang Y, *Sleep Medicine*, 2012–2014

'Pregnancy leads to long-lasting changes in human brain structure', Hoekzema E, Barba-Müller E, Pozzobon C et al. www.nature.com/articles/nn.4458 (2016)

'Could listening to music during pregnancy be protective against postnatal depression and poor wellbeing post birth? Longitudinal associations from a preliminary prospective cohort study', Fancourt D and Perkins R, *British Medical Journal* (2017)

'Language experienced in utero affects vowel perception after birth: a two–country study', Moon C, Larger crantz H and Kuhl PK doi.org/10.1111/apa.12098, (2012)

'How Consonants and Vowels Shape Spoken-Language Recognition', Nazz T and Cutler A, *Annual Review of Linguistics* (2019)

'Caffeine intake in pregnancy is associated with low birth weight: a systematic review and dose respondent meta analysis', Chen L et al, *BMC Medicine* (2014)

'Moderate caffeine consumption during pregnancy', *Committee Opinion*, American College of Obstetrics and Gynaecologists (2010 and reaffirmed 2016)

Diabetes UK www.diabetes.org.uk/Professionals/Position-statements-reports/Statistics

'Antenatal perineal massage for reducing perineal trauma', Beckmann MM and Garrett AJ, Cochrane Database of Systematic Reviews (2006)

'Perineal massage in labour and prevention of perineal trauma: a randomised controlled trial', Stamp G, Kruzins G and Crowther C, British Medical Journal (2001)

'Male symptoms: A critical review of the Couvade syndrome: The pregnant male', Brennan A, Ayers S, Ahmed H and Marshall-Lucette S, Journal of Reproductive and Infant Psychology, 25(3), pp. 173–189. (2007).

'Perineal outcomes and maternal comfort related to the application of perineal warm packs in the second stage of labor: a randomized controlled trial,' Dahlen HG, Homer CS, Cooke M, Upton AM, Nunn R, Brodrick B. (2007) www.ncbi.nlm.nih.gov/pubmed/18021143

'Episiotomy and perineal tears: Your pregnancy and baby guide' www.nhs.uk/conditions/pregnancy-and-baby/episiotomy/

'Antenatal care for uncomplicated pregnancies' NICE Guidelines: Clinical guideline [CG62], March 2008, Last updated: February 2019

'Systematic review of effects of low-moderate prenatal alcohol exposure on pregnancy outcome,' ObGyn Online, Henderson J, Gray R, Brocklehurst P (2007)

'Outcomes of Exercise Training Following the Use of a Birthing Ball During Pregnancy and Delivery', Fournier D, Feeney G, Mathieu ME, Journal of Strength and Conditioning Research July (2017)

'Effect of use of birthing ball on the first and second stage labour outcome among primigravidae', DCosta ID, Cutinho SP, International Journal of Nursing Education, (2015)

'Dads and PND: Sad dads. Paternal postpartum depression', Kim P, Swain JE, Psychiatry (Edgmont), (2007)

WHO Recommendations for Augmentation of Labour, Geneva, (2014) www.ncbi.nlm.nih.gov/books/NBK258883/

'Timing of Planned Caesarean Delivery by Racial Group', Balchin I, Whittaker JC, Lamont RF, Steer PJ FRCOG4, Obstetrics & Gynecology: March 2008, Volume 111, Issue 3, p 659–666

BMJ Clin Evid, Published online September 2008, 'Perineal care', Dr Chris Kettle and Susan Tohill

Seijmonsbergen-Schermers AE et al (2019). 'Which level of risk justifies routine induction of labor for healthy women?' *Sexual and Reproductive Healthcare,* doi.org/10.1016/j.srhc.2019.100479

'The Last Days of Pregnancy: A Place of In-Between', Jana Studelska, Mothering (2012) www.mothering.com/articles/the-last-days-of-pregnancy-a-place-of-in-between

'Melatonin Synergizes with Oxytocin to Enhance Contractility of Human Myometrial Smooth Muscle Cells', *J Clin Endocrinol Metab.* (2009 Feb); 94(2): 421–427. Published online 2008 Nov 11. doi: 10.1210/jc.2008-1723

Aromatherapy in Midwifery Practice, Denise Tiran, Singing Dragon, 2016

Compassion in practice, National Health Service Commissioning Board, Department of Health, London, (2012) www.england.nhs.uk/wp-content/uploads/2012/12/compassion-in-practice.pdf

'NICE stages of labour Intrapartum care for healthy women and babies', (2017) www.nice.org.uk/guidance/cg190/chapter/recommendations#latent-first-stage-of-labour

'Maternal positions and mobility during the first stage of labour', Lawrence A, Lewis L, Hofmeyr G, Styles C, Cochrane Database of Systematic Reviews (2013)

'What are the facilitators, inhibitors and implications of birth positioning? A review of the literature', Priddis H, Dahlen H, Schmied V. *Women and Birth* (2012)

'Position in the second stage of labour for women without epidural anaesthesia', Gupta JK, Hofmeyr GJ, Sood A, Vogel JP, Cochrane Database of Systematic Reviews (2017)

'Continuous support for women during childbirth', Bohren MA, Hofmeyr GJ, Sakala C, Fukuzawa RK, Cuthbert A, Cochrane Database of Systematic Reviews (2016)

'A Randomized Control Trial of Continuous Support in Labor', Campbell OA, Lake MF, Falk M and Backstrand JR, www.ncbi.nlm.nih.gov/pubmed/16881989

'Length of human pregnancy and contributors to its natural variation', Jukic et al, *Human Reproduction,* Vol.28, No.10 pp (2013)

NICE Inducing labour Clinical guideline [CG70] Published date: July (2008) www.nice.org.uk/guidance/cg70/chapter/4-Research-recommendations #prolonged-pregnancy

'Effect of Gravity on Placental Transfusion', *Lancet* 2:505–08. Yao AC and Lind J, (1969)

'Hypnosis for pain management during labour and childbirth', Madden K, Middleton P, Cyna AM, Matthewson M, Jones L (2016) www.cochrane.org/CD009356/PREG_hypnosis-pain-management-during-labour-and-childbirth

Birthplace study www.npeu.ox.ac.uk/birthplace (2011)

'Indigenous life stories: narratives of health and resistance. A dialogical narrative Analysis,' Blix BH, Hamran T and Normann HK *Canadian Journal of Nursing Research* Vol. 44 No 2, 64–85 (2012)

'Outcomes of planned home births and planned hospital births in low-risk women in Norway between 1990 and 2007: A retrospective cohort study' *Sexual & Reproductive Healthcare* Volume 3, Issue 4, Blix et al (2012)

'Continuous support for women during childbirth', Bohren MA, Hofmeyr GJ, Sakala C, Fukuzawa RK and Cuthbert A. Cochrane Database of Systematic Reviews (2017)

'Breastmilk-saliva interactions boost innate immunity by regulating the oral microbiome in early infancy', Al-Shehri Plos One (2015)

NICE: Postnatal care up to 8 weeks after birth, Clinical guideline [CG37] (2015)

'Pump Early, Pump Often: A Continuous Quality Improvement Project' *The Journal of Perinatal Education* Diane L. Spatz, Elizabeth B. Froh, Jessica Schwarz, Kathy Houng, Isabel Brewster, Carey Myers, Judy Prince, and Michelle Olkkola (2015)

'Neonatal recognition of the mother's face', I. W. R. Bushneil F. Sai J. T. Mullin, *British Journal of Developmental Psychology* (1989)

'Recognition of familiar faces by newborn' *Infant Behavior and Development*, Gail E.Walton, NJA Bower and TGR Bower (1992)

'The Impact of Adult Talk, Conversational Turns, and TV During the Critical 0–4 years of Child Development', *The Power of Talk*, 2nd Edition, Jill Gilkerson and Jeffrey A. Richards, (2009)

'Meaningful Differences in the Everyday Experience of Young American Children', Hart and Risley (1995)

'Managing infants who cry excessively in the first few months of life' Pamela Douglas, Peter Hill www.bmj.com/content/343/bmj.d7772 British Medical Journal (2011)

'Crying in Kung infants: A test of the cultural specificity hypothesis', Barr RG, Bakeman R, Konner M, Adamson L. Developmental Medicine and Child Neurology 33: 601–610. (1991)

'Systematic Review of Expected Weight Changes After Birth for Full-Term, Breastfed Newborns', Journal of Obstetric, Gynecologic & Neonatal Nursing Volume 48, Issue 6, Diane Di Tomasso and Mary Cloud (2019)

'The Biological significance of skin-to-skin contact and maternal odours', RH Porter, Acta Paediatrica (2004)

About the author

In 2012 Marie Louise qualified as one of the youngest midwives in the UK.

Whilst practising midwifery, she continued to study, and soon became a Band 6 midwife, also gained Level 3 Award in Education and Training (PTLLS) and a hypnobirthing diploma. She has travelled extensively across the USA and Asia to learn about midwifery in different cultures and has also lived and practised in Australia.

In 2019 she founded 'Modern Midwives Meet-ups', for like-minded professionals to share best practice and the latest research findings in an informal and relaxed setting.

What she imagined would be a get-together for a small group of midwives has become a national event that is hugely popular amongst some of the UK's leading birth experts.

'The Modern Midwife' on social media and the website has captivated a large audience of both midwives and expectant parents with her fun, informative and evidence-based posts. You can find them at: @the_modern_midwife and modernmidwife.com.

Marie Louise is a sought-after expert and has appeared live on *This Morning* and BBC *Woman's Hour* and has been invited to parliament to discuss maternal mental health and maternity discrimination.

Marie Louise always maintains: 'Being a midwife is not a job to me, it is part of who I am'. She has a clear focus on having the best possible impact on maternity's toughest challenges.

Acknowledgements

Even though I have wanted to write a book as far back as I can remember, never did I think my dream would come true and I would really be a published author. It has been ten years in the making, rather than the months it has taken to get on paper, and there have been many people that have been there along the way, helping me write this book.

Firstly, thank you to my family. When everyone told me I was too inexperienced and wouldn't get accepted into university (for such a mature job) my family told me to listen to my calling, ignore everyone else and apply.

To the university interviewers who saw, despite my age, I was meant to be a midwife.

My mentors, during my midwifery degree, for passing their wisdom and knowledge on so attentively. Especially **Joyce**; when I'd cry because I missed my family she always put an arm around me and told me how much of a great midwife I would be. From this support, I grew into a stronger woman, more able to stay on track and become the midwife I am today.

Every woman I have ever had the privilege of looking after at such an intimate, vulnerable and precious time of their life. Thank you for letting me learn about midwifery through each of your unique and individual experiences.

My **sister**, for always creeping around when I was on nights, and cooking food for me to wake up to when we lived together in Australia. You stood by me in my toughest times. My **brother**, who forever takes my stress and self-doubt away, for your lack of judgement and hilarious sense of humour lightening the solitude of writing. My **mum**, for all the hours you spent helping me write this book, making sure I knew it was achievable and doing anything I ever asked for. My hero, my **dad,** for revising every exam with me, always answering the phone and every question I have ever had with such logic and honesty. You picked me up when I started slipping into uncertainty about my ability and have shown me the meaning of unconditional love. My **partner** for travelling around the country with me for the midwives meetup events, never letting me think I wasn't good enough, for picking me up physically and mentally and for always making sure I was okay.

To **Sam Jackson** for believing in me as a writer, this book would not have happened without you. To **Laura Herring** and **Becky Alexander** for helping to crush my nerves and keeping me on track with your kind words and incredible editing skills. **Louise Evans** for your attention to detail and turning emails into beautiful illustrations.

Jason Foo for introducing me to **Fernando Desouches,** managing director at New Macho and for supporting me to write about how partners and men feel about pregnancy, birth and fatherhood.

Jess and **Michelle** you have been there through so much with me, so many phases both good and bad. 'It's just a test, you're being tested. Keep going.' I am eternally grateful for your excitement about this book, wise words and clarity when I felt overwhelmed.

My monk friend in Tibet, **Kan**, for welcoming me into your monastery, translating every conversation with patients, letting me sleep in your bed and showing me what selflessness really is. This book would not be the same without my experience with you.

To all the amazing women that have shared their birth stories, pearls of wisdom and support for other mums. You all inspired me: on the days when I didn't know where to start, I'd begin by reading your stories and then know what the book needed. I am so grateful for your time to write these out when you've got so much else to do.

My sistas, the midwives who also took time out of your equally busy lives to share your rich knowledge, you have been so supportive. We're one big team of modern midwives aiming at the same goal.

Candace Imison, Director of Strategy Development at the NMC, for your positive response to the book, your time to write a direct quote and for all of the work you are doing to 'Shape the Future NMC.'

Lastly, **Claire Mathews** and **Jaqueline Dunkly-Bent** for inviting me to shadow you, asking for my opinion and attentively listening to my answers. You are midwifery pioneers, full of modesty, and I hope I have made you proud.

Index

Page references in *italics* indicate images.

349

good mood food 269
GP 4, 6, 8, 9, 18, 23, 24, 72, 77, 78,
    79, 230, 231, 252, 262, 271, 301,
    309, 310
gratitude log 74–5, 77
green smoothies 55
Group B Strep (GBS) 200
gums, inflamed or bleeding 14–15
gut health 140, 269, 270–1, 286, 287

haemorrhoids (piles) 17, 120
hair ties 112
hand expressing 26–8, 230, 289
Hannah's story (birth story) 233–4
headaches 13, 53, 248
Healthy Baby Cohort Study, The, China
    (2012–2014) 20–1
'healthy' baby, idea of 163–4
Healthy Start scheme 53
heartbeat, baby's 33, 88, 89, 99, 211, 222,
    229, 274
heartburn 13, 17
Heidi's story (birth story) 234–7
help, asking for 324–5
Hepper, Peter 65
Hill, Millie 135
Hinckley, Marjorie Pay 144
Hindes, Katie 287
hip circling 117–18, 118
hip opener 119, 119, 120
HM Revenue and Customs (HMRC) 82
holding your baby 264, 264
holidays 15, 72, 89, 92
home birth 41, 94–6, 178, 231, 232, 241,
    244, 306, 307
home, creating in hospital 166–8
home handover 148
hormonal contraceptives 16
hormone hCG (Human Chorionic
    Gonadotropin) 8
hot water bottle/wheat bag 113
Hughes, Laura 50, 51–2, 139, 268
Hunter, Jemma 10–11, 14
hydration 9, 13, 15, 16, 19–20, 22, 53,
    72, 113, 154, 158, 204–5, 232, 248,
    268–9, 320
hydrotherapy 97
hyperemesis 8
hypnobirthing 19, 37, 70, 97, 113, 135,
    136, 178, 182, 186, 187, 193, 204,
    207, 209, 211, 228, 232, 233, 234–5

immunity 12, 268, 270–1, 286–8, 319
independent midwife (IM) 46–7
India, postnatal care in 255
induction of labour 39, 143, 145–6, 168,
    178, 230, 232, 233, 235, 236

inflammation 15, 264, 270, 286, 319,
    320–1, 322
information overload vii, 35–6, 329
injections 12, 98, 100, 101, 210
insomnia 20–1, 30, 271
Instagram ix–x, 14, 47, 109, 186, 252, 307,
    333
International Confederation of Midwives
    189–90

jasmine 167
jaundice 27, 277, 294
Jordan (birth story) 231–3

Kipling, Rudyard 87
Korte, Dianna 38

labour see birth
labour bag 110–14
lactoferrin 288
Lamb and Mango Coconut Curry 139–40
Lao Tzu 152
last menstrual period (LMP) 143
Laura (birth story) 229–31
lavender 19, 112, 138, 167, 203, 204, 257,
    258
learning in the womb, baby 63, 63, 64, 65, 79
let it go (acceptance) 72–5, 116
Lewis, Deborah 189–90
Liddell, Karni 163
lights, dimming the 168, 177
Lim, Melchor 312
linea nigra (line down your stomach) 15, 16
loneliness 28–9, 77, 91, 201, 279, 331
loose clothing 13

Make Birth Better 78, 309
Malaysia, postnatal care in 254
mammalian brain/reptile brain 174, 176,
    177, 187, 226
massage 16, 28, 97, 122–5, 123, 167,
    169–70, 169, 176–7, 193, 196, 221,
    233, 255, 256, 261, 281, 301, 320
Maternity Action 81
maternity discrimination 81–2
maternity knickers 114, 254
maternity leave 21, 79–80, 81, 151, 329
maternity pay 80, 81
Maternity Transformations Programme, The 46
Mathews, Claire 46
'Matrescence' 325
medication:
    birth and 97–9, 102, 164, 192, 196
    postnatal 230, 280, 314, 315
    pregnancy and 6, 18, 34, 72, 77, 78
meditation 5, 72, 77, 115, 204, 233, 234,
    320–1